One Minute Stress Management

NEW EDITION

FREEZE FRAME®

A Scientifically Proven Technique for Clear Decision Making and Improved Health

DOC CHILDRE

Edited by Bruce Cryer

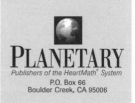

PLANETARY
Publishers of the HeartMath® System
P.O. Box 66
Boulder Creek, CA 95006

Published in the United States of America by:

Planetary Publications
P.O. Box 66, Boulder Creek, California 95006
(800) 372-3100 (831) 338-2161   Fax (831) 338-9861
info@planetarypub.com
http://www.planetarypub.com

Manufactured in the United States of America by BookCrafters.

First Edition 1994
Second Edition 1998

Jacket design by Abacus Graphics, Oceanside, CA

Library of Congress Cataloging-in-Publication Data

Childre, Doc Lew, 1945-
    Freeze-frame : one minute stress management : a scientifically proven technique for clear decision making and improved health / Doc Childre ; edited by Bruce Cryer.
        p. cm.
    Previously published with title: Freeze-frame, fast action stress relief : a scientifically proven technique.
    Includes bibliographical references.
    ISBN 1-879052-42-3
        1. Stress management--Popular works.   I. Cryer, Bruce.
II. Title
RA785.C448   1998
616.9'8--dc21   98-33558
                                                     CIP

                    10 9 8 7 6 5 4 3 2

"While managing a global video conferencing project at National Semiconductor, I had to coordinate a complex international team planning session. The results from using FREEZE-FRAME were absolutely phenomenal. We came back from our session knowing that we had achieved in two days what could have taken months had we not had this tool."

—Judith Hamilton, Videoconference Consultant

"...single most valuable, most effective and especially useful tool because people can do it in real time."

—Richard Podell, M.D.

"Breakthrough tools that make you more human, more effective and more balanced."

—Joseph Rende, Assistant Director of Educational Services for Global Research and Development, Young Presidents Organization

"My experience using IHM's FREEZE-FRAME technique to conquer my pre-TV appearance jitters was also enlightening. ...As I waited for my cue... I followed the instructions for FREEZE-FRAME. ...[My fear] receded to the edges of my awareness as surely as if I'd drawn an imaginary line in the sand of my consciousness... By the end of the interview, I was actually enjoying myself."

—*Country Living's Healthy Living*

A Note of Appreciation....

The second edition of *FREEZE-FRAME* includes the contributions of many friends, clients and supporters. Thanks to Donna Beech for her help in writing and shaping the new material, and her suggestions on design. Thanks to Dr. Alan Watkins for reading the manuscript and offering valuable suggestions. Several health professionals contributed invaluable tips and experience with FREEZE-FRAME: Dr. Pam Aasen, Dr. Joseph McCaffrey, Dr. Jeffrey Stevens, Dr. Greg Quinn, Dr. Bruce Wilson, Dr. Anne Berlin and Dr. Richard Podell. There were also many people who were willing to share their experience of improved health. Many thanks to the hundreds whose stories we didn't use and those whose we did: Patricia Chapman, Hobart Johnson, Joseph Chilton Pearce and Patrick Jacobs. Several of our clients and friends contributed stories that help illustrate the changes people experience: Vivian Wright, Victoria Hubbell, Lorie Russell, Emily Pendleton, Phyllis Gagnier, Lynn Marriot, Dennis Kelly, Jan Dawson and Vicky Tomasino. Thanks to the Institute of HeartMath's Rollin McCraty for helping to update the science chapter, and to Planetary's Sibyl Cryer for overseeing and organizing the project.

Table of Contents

Preface

Though FREEZE-FRAME technique has brought about incredible changes in people's lives since it was first introduced in the 1994 edition of this book. With just five simple steps, its effectiveness and impressive track record came as a surprise to some.

Because the technique was so simple, some people were amazed that it was being taught in many of the world's largest companies, on 35 U.S. military bases, was prescribed by medical doctors, and was successfully lowering conflict and raising performance with school children. They just found it hard to take FREEZE-FRAME too seriously. On the surface it was easy to perceive as a nice, little tool that was a lot like the visualization, focusing or breathing techniques used to control stress.

Although those techniques can be very helpful, there's a clear distinction between the FREEZE-FRAME process and other techniques. FREEZE-FRAME uses the power and intelligence of the heart to shift perception in the moment, bringing our biological systems, including the brain, into balance and harmony.

...there's a clear distinction between the FREEZE-FRAME process and other techniques. FREEZE-FRAME uses the power and intelligence of the heart to shift perception in the moment, bringing our biological systems, including the brain, into balance and harmony.

xi

The power of FREEZE-FRAME was brought to light through intensive biomedical research. Scientists at the Institute of HeartMath did numerous studies to understand the physiological effects of FREEZE-FRAME. They learned that when people practiced this technique, their heart rhythms changed, their nervous system became more balanced and, as a result, beneficial changes occurred in their hormonal patterns and immune system response. These biological changes added up to a significant shift in how we think and feel.

These amazing discoveries led to published research and increasing acceptance in the medical community. The Institute of HeartMath's (IHM) scientific studies have been presented at major medical and scientific conferences worldwide, and published in leading medical journals, such as *The American Journal of Cardiology, The American College of Cardiology, Stress Medicine* and *Journal for the Advancement of Medicine.*

Cardiologists, psychiatrists, psychologists and other physicians were excited to find an effective technique, backed by credible science, that could help their patients learn how to better shape their perceptions, overall behavior and health.

Expressing a common reaction of medical practitioners, Oakland, California cardiologist T. Gregory Quinn, M.D. said, "There are not many risk-free interventions. But this is one that has profound consequences. The implications of this are huge. Eighty percent of cardiology patients feel that stress is a major contributing factor to their disease. It's always been frustrating because historically there hasn't been much to offer them. Now there is."

FREEZE-FRAME became a core technology in HeartMath training programs and soon thousands of people in companies, government agencies, schools and hospitals were using the technique and experiencing great benefit. In organizational settings, people were finding FREEZE-FRAME highly useful, not only for improving health and managing stress, but also for making better decisions, enhancing creativity, and communicating and relating to others. Even more people were given access to FREEZE-FRAME through a video, an audiobook and various learning programs. Today thousands of individuals around the world have made FREEZE-FRAME a regular part of their lives.

With published research and successful implementation of FREEZE-FRAME, many in the media became intrigued with this simple technique that was clearly helping people in so many ways. Hundreds of television shows, magazines, newspapers and radio broadcasts in North America and the U.K. have now reported on and written about FREEZE-FRAME, and the interest continues to grow. We felt it was time to create this new edition to share all that has happened with FREEZE-FRAME and to update the scientific information that provides the underpinning for the technique. Doc also rewrote some of his original text and the book was reformatted to make it easier to follow. We have also included new stories from a variety of people who have been using FREEZE-FRAME. These stories are not intended to be promotional in nature or to convince you that the technique works, but rather to serve as examples of how you can apply FREEZE-FRAME in your life.

Enjoy this new edition of FREEZE-FRAME and become your own "self-scientist." By this I mean read and learn about FREEZE-FRAME and then try to apply the technique with sincerity. Hopefully, as others have, you will enjoy significant benefits from using these five simple steps to make decisions, solve problems, reduce stress and improve your health.

Howard Martin
President, Planetary LLC

Introduction

T he pressure's building. You feel so steamed up that your gauge has hit the danger zone and your lid is about to blow. It's been one thing after another today and you just can't take it anymore. You have to get away— take a walk on the beach, a hike in the mountains or a drive in the country.

Once you "get away from it all," you feel yourself begin to cool down and let a little steam out. Your racing mind begins to slow to a reasonable pace. As you look out across the landscape, you feel soothed and calm. You think back to your last vacation—how relaxed and energized you felt. That peaceful memory allows you to experience a shift in perspective.

While you were feeling the intense pressure, there seemed to be no way out, but now, in this relaxed state, things don't seem so bad. In fact, a few creative solutions that you hadn't thought of before start to seem like real possibilities. You realize how much more productive, creative and healthy you'd

Science has shown that we pay a serious price for our stress. *There is hope* because there is a solution. Recent scientific research has proven that you ·can learn not only to manage your stress, but even to prevent much of it before it happens. The key is within your *heart.*

xiv

be if you could have this same clarity and insight throughout the day—*even in the moments when stress is happening.*

Until recently, that might have been just wishful thinking, but since FREEZE-FRAME was first introduced, thousands of people have experienced just that—a more consistent state of high quality living, inner balance and reduced stress.

The world has become a pressure cooker with the burden of stress growing daily. One researcher has measured life as now 44% more difficult than in 1964. It's hard to ignore stress these days, especially with media reports constantly reminding you just how frightening and tough life has become—violence, drugs, floods, earthquakes, a decaying educational system, economic turmoil and the challenge of globalization. Your mind and emotions are bombarded daily with information that reinforces a perception of just how stressed you *should* feel. Even the statistics can be stressful:

- 75% to 90% of all doctor visits in the U.S. today are for stress-related disorders.[1]

- Job stress has become "the 20th century disease" and is considered a global epidemic.[2]

- Depression was the fourth leading cause of disease-burden in 1990 and by 2020 it will be the single leading cause.[3]

- The number of workers feeling highly stressed has doubled since 1985.[4]

- 61% of people surveyed in the U.S., U.K., Ireland, Germany, Singapore and Hong Kong believe information overload is present in their workplace, with 80% predicting the situation will worsen.[5]

■ "Karoshi"—death from overwork, is said by Japanese health activists to kill some 30,000 workers every year.[6]

■ Acute stress ("fight or flight" or major life events) and chronic stress (the cumulative load of minor, day-to-day stress) can both have long-term consequences.[7]

■ As much as 80% of all disease and illness (in the U. S.) is initiated or aggravated by stress.[8]

Science has shown that we pay a serious price for our stress. A twenty year study conducted by the University of London School of Medicine has determined that unmanaged mental and emotional reactions to stress present a more dangerous risk factor for cancer and heart disease than cigarette smoking or eating high cholesterol foods.

So, with a growing list of things to feel stressed about, what do you do? Fold up your tents and go home? Give your boss notice and not go back to work? Sell the car so you don't have to deal with rush hour traffic anymore?

The central message of this book is: *There is hope* because there is a solution. Recent scientific research has proven that you can learn not only to manage your stress, but even to prevent much of it before it happens. The key is within your heart. As you learn to *prevent* stressful reactions, you save a tremendous amount of energy—energy that can be used to develop creative projects, build fulfilling relationships, solve family problems, make more effective decisions and have more fun.

FREEZE-FRAME is also a powerful tool for creativity, innovation and problem solving. Creative thinking is an essential skill today with life's increasing complexity, data overload and time pressure. It's essential to keep the big picture in perspective, to be innovative and adaptive as the world changes. Being able to think "out of the box" has become a requirement for success in business, science or any creative endeavor. This implies a new kind of flexibility so that you can step back from your sense of overload or overwhelm and shift from a digital/logical mental process to intuitive heart intelligence.

Does that mean that if you learn this technique called FREEZE-FRAME, the boss will stop being so demanding, the company will reverse its decision to lay off 10% of the work force or your kids will suddenly turn into perfect angels? FREEZE-FRAME is not a quick fix for all of your problems. It is, however, a technique that can fix unnecessary stress quickly. Some things will change more quickly than others, but whatever life throws your way, you will have more strength, flexibility, common sense and insight to deal with it intelligently.

As you will see in the many stories and case studies throughout the book, these changes can have profound, positive implications for personal health, productivity, family fun, organizational coherence and a healthier, more intelligent society.

FREEZE-FRAME is the first tool in the HeartMath System. By learning this simple technique, you will strengthen your ability to make clear decisions and improve your health. You will learn how and why to listen to your heart to awaken more of your own intuitive intelligence. You'll hear about people who have transformed the quality of their lives and about organizations that function more creatively. And the next time you feel the pressure building—but there's no escape—you'll have a new solution. I invite you to try it out. It only takes a minute—a small price for a quality life with much less stress.

Taming the Stress Monster

> "The heart has had bad press. It's been hijacked by hearts-and-flowers stuff, yet it is the body's main power station and when we are in a positive emotional state, it can play a key role in balancing the entire human system, helping other organs to work together in harmony."
>
> Alan Watkins M.D., Author, *Mind-Body Medicine*

CHAPTER HIGHLIGHTS

- A Typical Stressful Day
- The Cost of Stress
- It's All About Perception
- The Purpose of FREEZE-FRAME

I t's been a typical day at the office for Nick. Too many interruptions. A staff meeting that went longer than planned. An additional two-week delay on a key product release. He is already running late to pick up his daughter Tracy from high school and the day's events are spinning in his mind. It hasn't been a terrible day really, just the usual time-crunch, stress and strain. As Nick pulls onto the freeway, there are more red tail lights staring at him than usual. "Damn! I'm going to be really late for Tracy."

Nick notices two lanes closed ahead for repaving. His mind and emotions race with frustration. Nick begins to remember all the unsolved problems from work, adding to his frustration, and triggering a sequence of physical changes inside his body. Unbeknownst to him, his emotional reaction is causing large amounts of adrenaline and the stress hormone cortisol to enter his bloodstream.

Nick's stress response is now in full gear. As the adrenaline reaches his heart, the heart begins to pound harder and harder. A little voice tells him to relax—"the traffic can't move until it moves"—but he ignores it and his frustration builds into resentment.

The excess adrenaline and cortisol are causing his immune system to shut down—not a good idea when you're under stress. The portion of his nervous system that normally would have calmed his heart is also shut down, so his heart keeps pumping out blood as though it were a life and death situation—more than he would ever need just sitting there in traffic. There are other effects too: sweaty palms, rapid breathing. All these physical responses send messages back to the brain reinforcing the perception of danger—drowning out the little voice that tells him to relax.

By now Nick is knee-deep in feeling victimized: "What a lousy day! When are they going to finish this freeway? Why can't my wife pick up Tracy?" The adrenaline, still going strong, causes yet another hidden effect in Nick. It is stimulating the release of fat cells into his bloodstream—he would have needed this extra energy if it had been a real emergency. Only it isn't. So, unbeknownst to him, his liver is converting the fat into cholesterol which is absorbed onto a scratch that just formed on his coronary artery. Some even gets stuck on the artery wall itself.[1]

Just then, the traffic starts to move and Nick heaves a huge sigh of relief. But the damage has been done. Drained and irritated, he jams down hard on the accelerator to race to his daughter's school, narrowly missing the side of an eighteen wheeler whose driver quickly lets him know how he feels about Nick's driving. Nick finally pulls up to the school where an impatient Tracy is in a phone booth calling to find out where dad is.

This all-too-common scenario gets replayed daily, with variations, all over the world. While some of the events in Nick's day are beyond his control, his responses could have been much different.

If he knew how to manage his emotional reactions to these events, Nick could have avoided the aggravation to his mood, his health and his family. The traffic wouldn't have moved any faster—and he may not have arrived at Tracy's school any sooner—but he could have alleviated his "inner" traffic jam and saved himself the energy drain, as well as the negative consequences to his health and well being.

The Cost of Stress

Stress stimulates the perpetual release of the hormones adrenaline, noradrenaline and cortisol, which eventually sear the body like a constant drizzle of acid. If left unchecked, chronic stress—along with attitudes like hostility, anger and depression—can sicken and eventually kill us. Here's what the latest studies have to say:

Heart Disease

⇨ According to a Mayo Clinic study of individuals with heart disease, psychological stress was the strongest predictor of future cardiac events, such as cardiac death, cardiac arrest and heart attacks. [2]

3

⇨ People with the highest allostatic load [stress] are most likely to develop cardiovascular disease and are significantly more likely to have declines in cognitive and physical functioning.[3]

⇨ A Harvard Medical School study of 1,623 heart attack survivors found that when subjects got angry during emotional conflicts, their risk of subsequent heart attacks was more than double that of those that remained calm.[4]

⇨ A 20-year study of over 1,700 older men conducted by the Harvard School of Public Health found that worry about social conditions, health and personal finances all significantly increased the risk of coronary heart disease.[5]

⇨ Heart disease cannot be explained by the standard risk factors—such as high cholesterol, smoking or sedentary lifestyle—in over half the cases.[6]

⇨ Heart disease, stroke and other circulatory diseases together kill more than 15 million people a year worldwide, or 30% of the annual total of deaths from all causes. [7]

⇨ Since 1984, more women have died each year of cardiovascular disease than men.[8]

⇨ Heart disease has led the list of killers in virtually every industrialized society for the past 30-40 years. Total economic cost for cardiovascular disease in the U.S. in 1998 (est.) is $274.2 billion. That's $15 billion more than in 1997. [8]

Hypertension

(sustained, elevated blood pressure)

⇨ An estimated 691 million people have high blood pressure, worldwide.[9]

⇨ Hypertension exists among approximately 60 million Americans.[8]

⇨ People who say they are feeling anxious or depressed are two to three times more likely to go on to develop high blood pressure than calmer, happier individuals.[10]

Death

⇨ Three 10-year studies concluded that emotional stress was more predictive of death from cancer and cardiovascular disease than smoking; people who were unable to effectively manage their stress had a 40% higher death rate than non-stressed individuals.[11]

⇨ Sudden cardiac death is up to 6 times more likely among men who complain of high anxiety than those who are calmer.[12]

⇨ Death rate per 100,000 women from coronary heart disease is three times greater than the death rate per 100,000 women from breast cancer (the disease women fear the most.)[8]

It's All About Perception

Research at the Institute of HeartMath shows that the amount of stress you feel is based more on your perception of a person, place or event, than on the event itself.

After the 7.1 earthquake in northern California in 1989, for example, the survivors had a wide range of reactions that were unrelated to the severity of their loss. In the following year, many people moved away from the state, determined to never go through such a terrifying experience again. Others needed therapy to speed the healing from their trauma. However, there were those who lost their homes yet adapted quickly and even expressed appreciation that the community had come together as a family, neighbors helping neighbors, the way life is supposed to be.

While natural disasters are dramatic, an unexpected change of any kind can be very stressful. Major life transitions—such as marriage, divorce, changing jobs, changing residence, children leaving home—test your capacity to adapt and remain flexible. Your ability to bounce back, pick up the pieces and move on with your life is directly related to your perception of what occurred. Those who recover most quickly and successfully are those who realize that, like it or not, they can't change what happened. Using their common sense, they adapt and move on with life as quickly as possible.

Learning how to FREEZE-FRAME means understanding how to choose our perceptions so they are the most healthful and productive possible, and gives us access to the "bigger picture" perspectives with new, creative opportunities and options.

The Purpose of FREEZE-FRAME

Why do I call it "FREEZE-FRAME"? When you watch a movie, what you are seeing is a series of still frames on film that are actually moving rapidly past the film projector's light source. Life can often seem like a high-speed movie that keeps getting faster without our knowing how to slow it down. How you *choose* to respond each moment to the movie of life determines how you see the next frame, and the next, and eventually how you feel when the movie ends. When you're mentally or emotionally reacting to life—with frustration, anxiety or indecision—you are releasing self-poisoning stress hormones into your system, draining your energy and distorting your perspective. Consequently, your next choice may not be an intelligent one. FREEZE-FRAME enhances the power to stop your reaction to the movie at any moment, call "time-out" and get a clearer perspective on how to adapt to what's happening on the screen. Instead of *self-poisoning*, you gain *self-poise*. Anyone can do it.

In the past you may have been told, "Stop and count to ten" or "Think positively." Or today you might hear an expression like "Chill." Counting to ten may help cool you down for a moment, but doesn't change your *perception* of the person or situation. Chances are, by the count of eleven, you've reengaged, and are caught up in the same emotional spiral.

Often people go to a quiet place, take a walk on the beach or go jogging when they need clarity. This too is a welcome escape, but still temporary, and often an impractical option. FREEZE-FRAME causes an immediate and profound shift in how you view the situation you are in, breaking the stress cycle by removing its source. By using your heart to shift your perception, it can work quickly right where you are. It's like bringing that walk on the beach right back to you in a moment—when you're rushing to meet a deadline or in a tense staff meeting or in an argument but can't get away to unwind—you can gain more peace and clarity *now!*

Have you noticed how swiftly life's events can change your moods? You could be walking down the street, feeling angry at something or someone. Suddenly the laughter and joy of a baby seizes your attention. You smile. Passing a favorite store, you spot a half-price sale going on, and the new leather jacket you wanted is on sale! Your whole mood shifts. Life's okay again even if you were in a bad mood a "frame" before.

Hormonally, you've changed too. You experience an obvious uplift as you make your purchase. On the way out of the store, you pass dozens of TVs on the wall. You're lured by the latest gruesome crisis being reported on CNN—live, as it's happening. Your mood crashes once more. FREEZE-FRAME is an opportunity to make on-the-spot attitude adjustments so life doesn't entrap you in an emotional roller coaster.

Kids are often more emotionally resilient than adults. They can be in a scuffle on the playground one minute, and be best friends again a few minutes later. It usually takes adults much longer to let go of emotions, because the developed adult mind has learned to replay the angry thoughts and feelings repeatedly. This habit depletes people from the inside-out.

When calming children down when they are hurt or upset, adults often get creative. You might remind them about something fun they're going to do tomorrow or assure them that the friend who just grabbed their toy is really a good person. You do this to help them release the emotional stress and calm down. As adults, we need a mature way to find that same stillness we're helping our children find. FREEZE-FRAME doesn't take the spice out of life; it gives us the opportunity to manage ourselves so the fun times can be even more fun, and the down times aren't so down.

Research has shown that it's the daily accumulation of little stresses that take more of a toll on your health than the major stressful events in life. How drained you are from the daily stresses also determines how much resilience you have when a real crisis occurs. Unless you learn to neutralize these reactions as they occur, they stack up and drain your health and clarity, leading to more compounded stress.

"Road rage" is a good example. Many people feel victimized by traffic before the work day has even begun. Traffic can make people feel frustrated, angry and resentful. These emotions, if not managed, can accumulate and explode in dangerous ways. FREEZE-FRAME won't free up the traffic lane. The traffic still won't move until it moves. But it will keep you from aging needlessly before the traffic moves, aggravating the other drivers, or storing up your traffic stress and then taking it out on people at work or home.

Flow

The great athletes or dancers can relax as they focus on what they're doing—finding a flow and rhythm with it. Higher performance is invariably the result. With the FREEZE-FRAME technology, you learn to employ that exact principle with any task or mental and emotional activity.

Have you ever watched an intense game of basketball where Team A senses they're losing their "cool" because Team B is "in sync" and is running away with the game? Team A calls a time-out. Why? Because Team A knows that:

- If they slow things down for a couple of minutes, they can obtain a clearer perspective of what's happening and start functioning better as a team.

- They can formulate some quick adjustments to attempt to switch the momentum back to their side.

- They can take time-out to recover lost energy and recharge.

- They can regain their composure after feeling "victimized" by how well Team B was playing. The coach can encourage them to "go for it" and put more heart into their playing.

These same reasons for taking a time-out in the game apply to your life right now in this moment. You could look at all the players of the team as a single energy unit, like the human body. When you regroup and FREEZE-FRAME in the heart, your entire system—glands, organs and nervous system—begins to work as a complete unit, yielding more available energy.

Let's discuss the steps of this time-out process. If you already practice a similar technique, read on anyway. You'll be able to appreciate the scientific verification and probably discover new applications from this technology.

The Five Steps of FREEZE-FRAME

1. Recognize the stressful feeling and FREEZE-FRAME it! Take a time-out.

2. Make a sincere effort to shift your focus away from the racing mind or disturbed emotions to the area around your heart. Pretend you're breathing through your heart to help focus your energy in this area. Keep your focus there for 10 seconds or more.

3. Recall a positive, fun feeling or positive time you've had and attempt to reexperience it.

4. Using your intuition, common sense, and sincerity—ask your heart, what would be a more efficient response to the situation, one that will minimize future stress?

5. Listen to what your heart says in answer to your question.

Five minutes out of your day can save you hours of turmoil, reactivity and just plain, unproductive time!

11

Let's explain these five steps in more detail.

STEP ONE

Recognize the stressful feeling and FREEZE-FRAME it! Take a time-out.

You have to realize you're experiencing stress before you can stop it. In addition to the chemical fireworks going off inside your body, most people also develop tension in their muscles when they're under stress. Do your shoulders get tight? Does your stomach get queasy? Does your head start to ache? Do you forget where you were going or what you were doing? Do you get abrupt with people or take everything personally? Learn to recognize your cues for stress. Then FREEZE-FRAME. Recognizing stress gives you the opportunity to do something about it!

Once you've recognized it, take a time-out. Acknowledge that you need a new perspective and step back from the problem. It's like pushing the pause button on your VCR. If you don't take time out for a moment or two, you'll never really be able to look carefully and objectively at what is needed to make the most effective decision. Think about it this way: If you want to be the director of your own movie, you have to stop being just one of the characters and step back to see the whole picture.

At first, you may not catch yourself until after the stress reaction has occurred. Your headache is already in full bloom. You've already snapped at your coworker. It may be a little late, but recognizing the stress "after the fact" is a whole lot better than not at all. Many people process negative thoughts and feelings for hours, days, weeks, months, and longer.

Learning how to shorten the time you spend on all that unnecessary stress is what FREEZE-FRAME is about. Each time you practice, you'll get faster and more proficient.

STEP TWO

Make a sincere effort to shift your focus away from the racing mind or disturbed emotions to the area around your heart. Pretend you're breathing through your heart to help focus your energy in this area. Keep your focus there for 10 seconds or more.

By shifting focus to the heart and away from the problem, you remove energy from your perception of the problem. This allows you to consider more effective possibilities.

Imagine a stressed-out person who's car gets stuck in the mud. Panicking, he stomps on the gas pedal. His tires spin wildly, sinking deeper and deeper into the murk. He's not going to get himself free that way. If he could step back, FREEZE-FRAME, and find a calm, objective view of the situation, he'd access more clarity. With clarity you can frame strategies and solutions that are productive and that you feel good about later. You also save personal energy and aging with this self-initiated effort.

When I say to focus your attention around the area of your heart, you might ask, is that just a convenient way to distract the mind or is there more to it? There's a lot more! Attention shifting is common in many practices. Meditation

☑ **If you are having difficulty shifting your attention to the area around the heart, first focus on your left big toe, wiggle it and see how it feels and how easy it is to redirect your attention. Now, shift your focus to the area around your heart. You can pretend to breathe through your heart or hold your hand over your heart to help focus your attention in this area. Keep your focus here for 10 seconds or more.**

13

involves shifting your attention to a mantra, sound or your breath. What's important in FREEZE-FRAME is that you are shifting to the heart. This emphasis on the heart is not just metaphorical. Expressions like, "She speaks from the heart" and "He played with all his heart" are now being verified in the research lab. In the next chapter, you'll learn how shifting your focus from head to heart boosts cardiovascular efficiency and enhances communication between heart and brain, bringing more coherence to the mind and emotions.

STEP THREE

Recall a positive, fun feeling or positive time in life and attempt to reexperience it.

Examples could be a fun, relaxing vacation; the love you feel for a child, spouse or parent; a moment you spent in nature; the appreciation you feel for someone or something in your life. Remember the *feeling*, such as joy, appreciation, care, compassion or love. In the lab, it's been shown that experiencing these positive feelings provides regeneration to the immune system, facilitating health and well-being. And these positive feelings can assist you in seeing the world with more clarity, discernment and balance.

What's important to remember in this step is to reexperience the *feeling*. It's not just mental visualization—where you simply picture something in your mind. For instance, if you use your great vacation in Hawaii to trigger a positive feeling, you may remember the moonlight shining on the water or the wind gently blowing through the palm trees as you stood on the beach in front of your hotel. But don't stop there. What did that experience *feel* like—not just what it looked like? This step is intended to evoke the feeling memory.

Experiencing a positive feeling can be difficult at times, especially if the situation you are now in is extremely stressful and emotionally charged. But the effort made to shift focus to a feeling like appreciation, whether from the past or in the present, helps you *neutralize* the negative reaction.

Even if you aren't able to experience feelings of appreciation, care or compassion, at least try to become neutral. Becoming neutral in the face of stress is major progress compared to the consequences of ongoing emotional drain. Finding a neutral state facilitates hormonal balance, releasing the aggressive mental and emotional stress reactions. From neutral you have options on how to proceed. It helps take the stress monkey off your back by unclouding your mind and emotions. This keeps you from judging and reacting too quickly and paying the stress tax later.

Richard Podell, M.D., an internist and clinical professor in Family Medicine at the University of Medicine and Dentistry of New Jersey, and certified FREEZE-FRAME trainer, has used and taught FREEZE-FRAME for about 2 1/2 years. Dr. Podell has trained in group settings as well as over one hundred individual patients, who typically "can learn to do it in two one-hour sessions." He says that once the patient has identified the image, experience or person that triggers feelings of appreciation, care or love, the process becomes clear and easy to do and they get great results.

While he has integrated stress management into his practice for the past 15 years, he describes FREEZE-FRAME as the "single most valuable, most effective and especially useful tool because people can do it in real time. FREEZE-FRAME can be done anywhere without anyone else having to know that you're doing it!"

Cardiologist Bruce Wilson, M.D., is introducing FREEZE-FRAME as a formal component in the Cardiac Rehabilitation program at his hospital in Milwaukee, Wisconsin. One of the many patients to whom Dr. Wilson has given a *FREEZE-FRAME* book told him, "When I was in Vietnam, we were lying in the trenches, scared all the time. We thought we were going to die every day. But there was this one morning in particular, when the sun came up—brilliant orange—and I could see through the trees. And just for a second, I was so glad to be alive. When I do a FREEZE-FRAME, I remember that wonderful, relaxed feeling. That's what comes to me every time I do this."

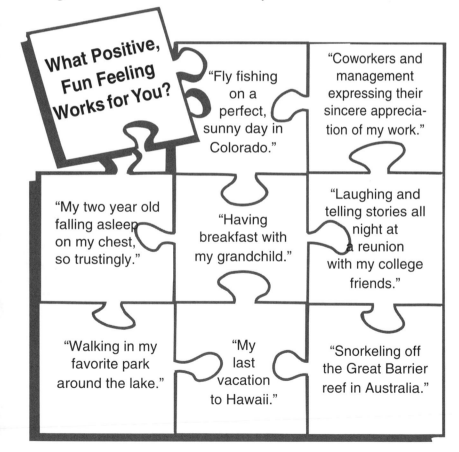

STEP FOUR

Now, using your intuition, common sense and sincerity— ask your heart, what would be a more efficient response to the situation, one that will minimize future stress?

As you practice FREEZE-FRAME, your intuition, common sense and sincerity will become more active and available. While you won't necessarily have crystal-clear insights every time you FREEZE-FRAME, you can at least increase your capacity to arrive at convenient and practical solutions.

With the guidance of your heart, you can make quality decisions and your life will be more fun. Being alive in the heart is what makes life worthwhile. When you are in touch with your heartfelt emotions, you find your true core values and enrich your life. The mind operating without the heart can create conveniences in the moment which, without heart direction, can generate stress later. It's the harmonious joint venture between the heart and mind that brings people quality experience in work, play and especially in relationships.

As you practice this step, stay focused in the area around the heart as you sincerely ask the question. This will keep you anchored so you don't jump right back into the stress loop of mismanaged emotions.

STEP FIVE

Listen to what your heart says in answer to your question. (It's an effective way to put your reactive mind and emotions in check—and an in-house source of common-sense solutions!)

Once the noise of your mind and emotions is quieted, you can hear what some call the "still, small voice." Finding this inner wisdom or intuition requires making a shift, like changing the radio setting from AM to FM. As your system becomes more "coherent," the brain begins to synchronize with the heart, cortical facilitation occurs and more power and intelligence become available to the brain. This results in a shift in perception and access to new information that before could have seemed fuzzy or vague.

Sometimes the answers you arrive at through FREEZE-FRAME can be very simple, or perhaps verification of something you already know. Other times you may experience a download of new information and fresh perspectives. At other times, you may not get a clear answer at all, but more often than not you will experience a shift in perception. What's important here is that you make an effort to follow your heart's directive.

Here is a brief essence of FREEZE-FRAME:

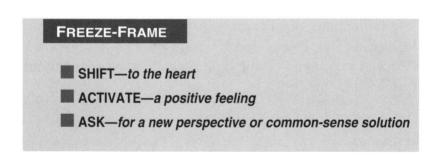

Practice—Applying the Steps

Practicing FREEZE-FRAME is easier than you may think. It's a process that many people already do naturally on occasion. The intelligence of pausing to take a deeper look before making decisions is already inherent within the heart of each person. You can learn to calm and manage the mind and emotions before making choices in day-to-day life. When you act from a point of balance, it results in increased mental and emotional poise. This eliminates stress on contact and connects you with what your real self would think or do.

Practice is not work; it's something that works for you. As you see the results, it becomes fun. Fun "eats" stress, just like the video game character, "Pac Man." Going through the steps one at a time will help you find a new perspective that can reduce or prevent your stress. Don't expect miracles or perfection. Skill is developed over time through sincere effort. It's the lack of sincerity that inhibits efforts from reaching their mark.

When I was learning to drive a car, before I could coordinate the clutch, brake and accelerator pedal, I'd use the brake to slow down and stop the car without pressing the clutch. There was a lot of clunk and clank in my ride until I remembered to use the clutch. I realized I was putting a lot of strain on the car and creating embarrassing situations—like lurching out into the middle of an intersection while the stoplight was changing.

FREEZE-FRAME is like putting the clutch in, allowing the flywheel (your emotions) to disengage, and giving you options of shifting gears, using the brakes or both. When you're in turmoil and attempt to apply the brakes to your emotions, that suppresses them and places a lot of wear and tear on your system. FREEZE-FRAME helps you get off the accelerator. You don't have to shut the car off (as in repressing yourself—that's not good for you either). You just shift the car into neutral and balance the emotions, allowing your mind to comprehend more fully what options you really have.

Pitfalls and Tips

When you start learning any new skill, program or sport, there are always potential pitfalls such as discouragement, not having the time to practice or simply forgetting to do it. Whether you're a business person, truck driver, teacher, parent or student, it's easy to get entangled in the daily routine of life. Having to remember to do something new requires sincere, self-initiated efforts. As you've read, the potential benefits of Freeze-Framing for improved health, vitality, performance and well-being are numerous. That's motivation number one. It's you taking care of you. Once you start to practice, it becomes smoother and easier, as with any skill. Before long, your common sense will help you remember.

As you feel better and see your intuition become more accessible through Freeze-Framing, you'll be propelled to continue using this tool. That's motivation number two. Freeze-Framing is very different from "Stop and take a deep breath" or "Stop and count to 10," because those techniques can be just the mind counting, which may not expand perception at all. That's why the intent of Freeze-Framing is to bring your energies to your heart. As the research in Chapter 3 describes, activating the power of the heart provides physiological benefits along with increased mental and emotional clarity. The step-by-step FREEZE-FRAME technique leads you to positive feelings that empower intuitive perception. Each FREEZE-FRAME step is important: to neutralize stress, activate the power of the heart and achieve new insight.

The best way to begin to practice FREEZE-FRAME is with little stresses that occur—traffic jams, things that aggravate you, problems at work. Some people forget to exercise their FREEZE-FRAME muscle until there's a major crisis. Since they haven't built their inner strength on smaller problems, they become discouraged if the technique doesn't immediately solve a "big one." Start small—one step at a time. You don't have to shy away from using FREEZE-FRAME on the big stressors; just remember you're building an inner muscle and that takes time. Practicing on small irritations, frustrations and disappointments as they happen will give you the encouragement and confidence to FREEZE-FRAME when weightier problems arise.

You won't have to FREEZE-FRAME all your life. The whole purpose and design of this one-minute technique is to take you into an automatic process. Then it's just you managing your energies the way people are naturally capable of anyhow. Regular practice of the technique is valuable because it facilitates the process of remembering until it's automatic. Then you will be able to activate the power inherent within you with continuity.

FREEZE-FRAME Exercise

1. Think of a current stressful situation in your life and write down a few words about it on the FREEZE-FRAME Worksheet on page 22. Don't pick the biggest, most emotionally-charged example yet.

2. Where it says **"head reaction,"** write down what you've been going through—feeling mad, worried, anxious, impatient, frustrated, burned out—whatever you've been thinking and feeling. *By "head," we mean the combination of mind and emotions without the heart involved.*

3. Take a minute to review the steps. Now relax, close your eyes if you like and go through the steps. (While you're learning, closing your eyes makes it easier to learn how to shift perception. Once you get the knack of it, you can FREEZE-FRAME with eyes open or closed.) When you're ready, write your heart answer under **"intuitive perspective."**

FREEZE-FRAME WORKSHEET

Current stressful situation:

_____

_____

_____

_____

Head Reaction:

_____

_____

_____

_____

FREEZE-FRAME IT!!

1. Recognize the stressful feeling and FREEZE-FRAME it! Take a time-out.

2. Make a sincere effort to shift your focus away from the racing mind or disturbed emotions to the area around your heart. Pretend you're breathing through your heart to help focus your energy in this area. Keep your focus there for 10 seconds or more.

3. Recall a positive, fun feeling or time you've had in life and attempt to reexperience it.

4. Now, using your intuition, common sense and sincerity, ask your heart—what would be a more efficient response to the situation, one that will minimize future stress?

5. Listen to what your heart says in answer to your question.

Intuitive Perspective:

_____

_____

_____

_____

_____

_____

_____

_____

_____

_____

© 1995 Institute of HeartMath

Now look at your FREEZE-FRAME worksheet. Read what you wrote under "head reaction," and then read what you wrote under "intuitive perspective." Is there a difference? If so, describe the difference you see as follows:

Find one or two words that capture the essence of the head reaction, such as "angry," "emotional" or "impatient." Now find one or two words that describe the intuitive perspective, such as "calm," "logical" or "caring." Then write them in below.

EXAMPLE

Someone may FREEZE-FRAME about a situation and shift from "confusion to clarity" or from "anger to acceptance."

In doing the FREEZE-FRAME exercise,
I shifted from_____to_____

For the next few weeks, practice the steps 4 or 5 times a day. "But, what if I don't have 4 or 5 things to FREEZE-FRAME?" you might ask. If you truly do the first step and learn to recognize stress, you'll discover many situations to apply FREEZE-FRAME to throughout the day. Remember the little things. Minor irritations—a subtle feeling of impatience, a moment of confusion—can all be shifted to a more coherent, creative perspective.

Practice FREEZE-FRAME prior to situations that could turn stressful—phone calls, meetings, prioritizing projects, picking up your teenager at school, other personal situations. FREEZE-FRAME is a powerful method to *prevent* stress before it has a chance to accumulate and drain your vitality.

A Job for FREEZE-FRAME

Let's say you need a new car and have a strict budget—about $18,000. You have a car in mind and go to the dealership to select it. But as you walk into the showroom, you see the car of your dreams! It has enough bells and whistles that the car within your budget now looks undernourished and wimpy. Suddenly, you're overwhelmed by mobile lust. The price tag? $40,000.

Your heart says, "This is crazy, but maybe in a year or so." Your mind says, "I couldn't make the payments, but what if I gave up aerobics, eating out, designer underwear and my paid vacation! (I'll take the pay but won't vacate)." Again your heart says, "Just say no!" But your mind is dazzled, victimized by the clutches of the showroom's glamour. Once again your heart insists, "It would be too much of a stretch to make payments..." Then, appropriately, along comes the car dealer, who says, "If you take the dream car today, I'll knock $2,000 off the price and give you a good deal on a trade-in." That does it! All the justification you needed. Like most people, you love to buy anything you can get "on sale." You decide to buy the "car of your dreams." After all, it was on sale!

Friend, right then is when you could use the convenience of a FREEZE-FRAME. Why? Because your heart's intuitive common sense said "no" to the expensive car of your dreams, but your mind fell vulnerable to the glitter—and the sale! A FREEZE-FRAME could be your last chance to steer your mind back into the real world. You could save those years of extra stress and aging by not buying your dream car until you were financially able to afford it. The novelty of that expensive car will likely wear off in a few months. However, those oversized payments and the accompanying stress can go on and on and on. Discover FREEZE-FRAME and give yourself a last chance to listen to your heart before you engage in an unnecessary, stressful commitment. You can preserve your mental and emotional health and peace by preventing these types of impulses.

This is a graphic example of the convenience of a FREEZE-FRAME. I'm sure you can backtrack and consider similar situations in your past—times when just *one* FREEZE-FRAME could have provided you deeper insight before you leaped into a decision which brought you months or even years of repeated stress. This story illustrates the inner self-talk we often have. Practicing FREEZE-FRAME regularly helps you remember to use the technique at major, decision-making crossroads.

I could tell you story after story about myself, when I reacted too quickly, without inner poise or clarity. The taxes I paid on those inefficient reactions motivated me to find an internal, decision-making tool that could bring me clarity before acting. In searching for such a tool, I had to take a closer look at how I arrived at decisions. I saw that there were two aspects of myself repeatedly in conflict—which I termed the head and the heart. There had to be an avenue for balancing my mental (or emotional) impulses with my core intuitive feelings. I experienced those core feelings occasionally, and noticed they seemed to bring the clarity I needed. I wanted to understand the inner mechanics of my head and heart so I could regularly access that core intuition. Through observing my inner self-talk, I saw that when I could really calm my head thoughts and emotions, then my core intuitive feelings became more clear. I began to develop the technique of FREEZE-FRAME and taught the steps to others to see if they'd have the same results. When they did, I decided to scientifically research what was occurring in the heart and brain while someone Freeze-Framed. Since people also reported improved health after regularly practicing FREEZE-FRAME, the scientists I was working with wanted to test what effect this technique was having on the immune system as well. The results were especially encouraging. FREEZE-FRAME proved to be a simple technique that puts the heart, mind, brain and emotions in a resonant state, creating the inner atmosphere for intuitive clarity.

Let's take a look at the scientific basis for FREEZE-FRAME.

The Scientific Basis of FREEZE-FRAME

Chapter 3

CHAPTER HIGHLIGHTS

- Heart Rate Variability
- The Electrical Heart
- Heart Hormones and the Immune System

FREEZE-FRAME is a tool whose effectiveness has been scientifically substantiated in a variety of research studies. The implications of this research are profound. People have long searched for a pill, drug or device that would give them better health or happiness. In the USA, 8 of the 10 top-selling prescription drugs are for stress-related problems[1], such as ulcers, hypertension, depression and anxiety. Science is proving that dependency on these drugs can lead to additional stress from side effects or addiction.

New research is proving what many of us already knew intuitively—that your mental and emotional attitudes directly affect your health.

The Research Division of the Institute of HeartMath is showing how and why our mental and emotional attitudes have such profound effects on the heart's electrical system and on the immune and hormonal systems.

It's important to realize that the flourishing sales of these prescription drugs are dwarfed by astronomical sales of illegal drugs that millions take in the pursuit of feeling better—drugs like cocaine, heroin and crack. According to the Mayo Clinic, in the past decade cardiovascular fitness has become synonymous with good health. New research studies on the heart are being released at a rapid rate. The Research Division of the Institute of HeartMath is engaged in several areas of investigation showing how and why our mental and emotional attitudes have such profound effects on the heart's electrical system and on the immune and hormonal systems. This research is proving what many of us already know intuitively—that our mental and emotional attitudes are directly related to our health and happiness.

The Role of the Heart

In addition to being an efficient pump supplying blood to our entire body, the heart is also our main electrical power center. Producing 2.5 watts of power, it generates 40 to 60 times more electrical power than the brain. The heartbeat, which produces an electrical signal, can be measured at any point on the body. A doctor could place electrodes on your ear lobes, little toe or anywhere on your body and record your electrocardiogram (ECG) signal. Quite literally, the electrical signal from the heart permeates every cell and, in fact, studies at the HeartMath research center are showing that the quality of that signal can affect your cells.

Heart Rate Variability—A Key Measure of Mental and Emotional Balance

If you go to a doctor's office for a physical exam, you may be told your heart is beating at 70 beats per minute. This is an average figure because the time intervals between heartbeats are always changing, meaning your heart rate is always changing. Heart rate variability (HRV) is a measure of these beat-to-beat changes in heart rate as the heart speeds up and slows down in different patterns. These heart rate changes are influenced by almost anything the brain and mind process, such as thoughts and sounds, but they are especially influenced by your emotions.

There is a two-way communication system between the heart and the brain that regulates heart rate and blood pressure[2] and it is the interaction of signals flowing between the two that causes the heart rate to vary with each beat. Analysis of HRV is used by doctors to measure the balance between the sympathetic and parasympathetic nervous systems, two important branches of this communication system. Your thoughts, perceptions and emotional reactions are transmitted from the brain to the heart via these two branches of the autonomic nervous system and can be seen in the patterns of your heart rhythms.[3] See Figure A on the following page.

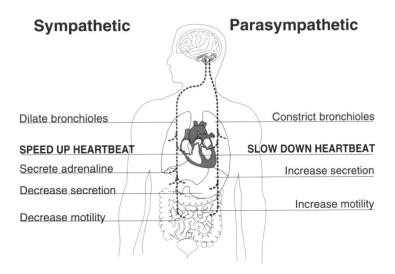

Sympathetic　　　　　　　　**Parasympathetic**

Dilate bronchioles　　　　　　　　　Constrict bronchioles

SPEED UP HEARTBEAT　　　　　　**SLOW DOWN HEARTBEAT**

Secrete adrenaline　　　　　　　　　Increase secretion

Decrease secretion

　　　　　　　　　　　　　　　　Increase motility

Decrease motility

Figure A. Your Nervous System
Simplified diagram of the autonomic nervous system. The sympathetic
branch increases heart rate and the secretion of adrenal hormones,
etc., whereas the parasympathetic slows heart rate and has a relaxing,
protective role. Proper function and balance between the two branches
of the ANS is important for good health.

The graph in Figure B(1) shows the typical HRV pattern of
someone feeling frustrated or edgy. When you feel edgy inside,
you are likely to experience this type of heart rhythm. This
excess wear and tear can create a chain reaction in your body.
For example, when you're frustrated, your nervous system is
out of balance, your blood vessels constrict, blood pressure
rises and you waste a lot of energy. If this happens consistently,
you can become hypertensive and greatly increase your risk of
heart disease. Hypertensive individuals are two to three times
more likely to develop coronary artery disease and four times
more likely to suffer a stroke. As you've already read, it's estimated that one in four Americans, approximately 60 million
people, are hypertensive.

Heart disease now accounts for slightly more than 40% of all deaths reported in the U.S.[4]

Figure B(1). Stress-Producing Heart Rhythm

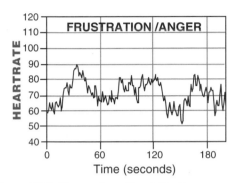

Time (seconds)

Figure B(2). Harmonious Heart Rhythm

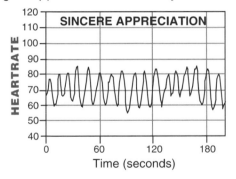

Time (seconds)

Figure B illustrates the heart rate variability pattern of frustration or anger *(top)* which is characterized by its random, jerky pattern. Sincere, positive feeling states like appreciation *(bottom)* can result in highly ordered and coherent HRV patterns, generally associated with enhanced cardiovascular function.

On the other hand, feelings of sincere appreciation create the HRV pattern you see in Figure B(2), which is a smooth, even rhythm. This pattern is an example of cardiovascular efficiency. What's happening is that the two branches of the autonomic nervous system are "entraining" and working together at maximum efficiency instead of fighting each other.

Think of entrainment as being "in sync." When your head and heart, thoughts and feelings, are working harmoniously together, you have more clarity and inner balance—and you feel better.

Another very important part of the heart/brain communication link are the nerves that carry information from the heart to the brain (see Figure C).

It is now known that the heart has a complex nervous system, which has been described as a "brain" of its own.[5] Considered a single entity, the brain in the heart is an organized network of nerve cells and nerve plexi (centers) that send messages to each other using neurotransmitters and proteins. The heart has a complex circuitry that enables it to act independently, learn, remember, and as the saying goes, produce the feelings of the heart. The brain in the heart plays a major role in human happiness or misery.

The information sent from the heart to the brain can have profound effects on the higher brain centers and influences perception, emotion and learning abilities. It even affects coordination and reaction speeds. IHM research shows that the FREEZE-FRAME process of focusing attention in the area of the heart while experiencing a positive feeling changes the patterns of information flowing along this pathway to a more coherent and harmonious pattern. This may explain the shift in perception experienced after Freeze-Framing. In addition to these perceptual shifts, many people have also been able to reduce their blood pressure and stress symptoms such as sleeplessness, indigestion and tension.[6]

Heart rate variability is an excellent measure of nervous system balance, and research is showing that your perceptions and reactions affect your heart rhythms [3,7]. Therefore, heart rate variability is an important indication of how well you are balancing your life.

Heart to Brain Communication System

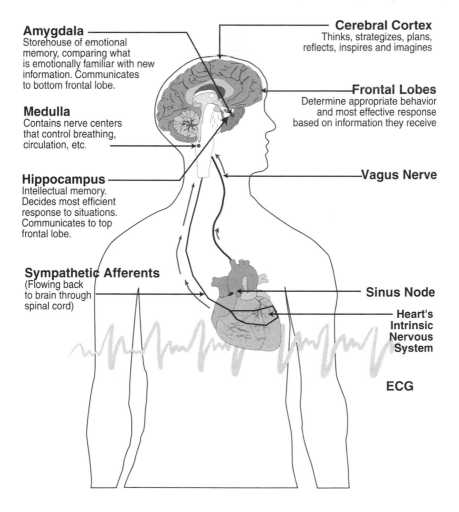

Amygdala
Storehouse of emotional
memory, comparing what
is emotionally familiar with new
information. Communicates
to bottom frontal lobe.

Cerebral Cortex
Thinks, strategizes, plans,
reflects, inspires and imagines

Medulla
Contains nerve centers
that control breathing,
circulation, etc.

Frontal Lobes
Determine appropriate behavior
and most effective response
based on information they receive

Hippocampus
Intellectual memory.
Decides most efficient
response to situations.
Communicates to top
frontal lobe.

Vagus Nerve

Sympathetic Afferents
(Flowing back
to brain through
spinal cord)

Sinus Node

**Heart's
Intrinsic
Nervous
System**

ECG

Figure C. Heart to Brain Communication System
The human body has hundreds of sensory systems which send
information back to the brain. The heart communicates to the brain via
two primary pathways.

As you become practiced in FREEZE-FRAME, you can balance your nervous system and change your heart rhythm patterns in the moment, as shown in Figure D.

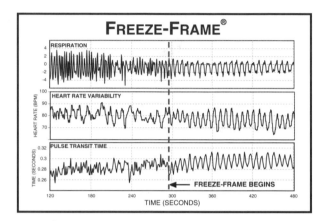

Figure D. Physiological Benefits of FREEZE-FRAME
These graphs show an individual's heart rate variability, pulse transit time and respiration patterns for 10 minutes. At the 300 second mark, the individual Freeze-Framed and all three systems came into entrainment, meaning the patterns are harmonious instead of scattered and out-of-sync.

Electrocardiogram Analysis

Besides looking at heart rate variability patterns, doctors also analyze electrocardiograms (ECG) to determine the health of the physical heart. For some years, scientists have been able to see the effects of hostility[8] and severe depression in the ECG.[9] Only recently, through the use of ECG spectral analysis, have they been able to see the effects of even more subtle "negative" emotions, such as frustration, worry and anxiety, as well as the effects of "positive" emotions such as love, care, compassion and appreciation.[3]

34

It is probably no coincidence that the electrical pattern of frustration in Figure E(1) looks about like it feels. When life is crashing down around you—your boss is yelling, pressure is mounting, the phone is ringing, the copier is jammed and you're frustrated—your ECG spectrum is likely to look like Figure E(1). This is called an "incoherent spectrum" and you probably feel pretty incoherent when life is falling apart.

Figure E(1) shows the spectrum analysis of eight seconds of electro-cardiogram (ECG) data generated by the heart when a person experiences *frustration or anger.* This is called an **incoherent spectrum** because the frequencies are scattered and disordered. **Figure E(2)** shows the frequency analysis of the ECG during a period when the person is experiencing deep, sincere *appreciation.* This is called a **coherent spectrum** because the power is ordered and harmonious.

Figure E(1). ECG: Incoherent Spectrum

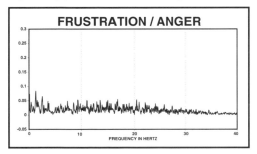

Figure E(2). ECG: Coherent Spectrum

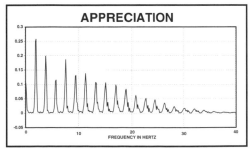

At other times, if your boss has just sincerely thanked you for a job well done, or you have a productive meeting with a coworker, or when you love what you're doing and feel appreciation for life, your ECG spectrum probably looks more like the harmonious pattern of Figure E(2), called a "coherent spectrum." At these moments, life is going your way and you feel more coherent—you have more clarity and balance. Feelings of love, care or compassion can all lead to a more coherent ECG spectrum, similar to the graph of appreciation. On the other hand, research has found that feelings of anger, anxiety, irritation or resentment all produce incoherent spectra that look similar to the graph of frustration. Remember, this electrical energy is being radiated to every cell in your body.

How Your Heart Affects Others

The electrical waves of the heart act like radio waves and are transmitted outside the human body as well as to every cell of your body. This may explain why you can sometimes walk into a room and tell if two people just had an argument, even though they are quietly standing there. You can "feel it in the air." The electrical frequencies radiated by the heart change dramatically when you are in different emotional states and can affect not only yourself but the people around you. In fact, the researchers at IHM have shown that the field radiated by your heart is literally picked up by the brains of people nearby! When two people are touching or even standing near each other, it is now possible to measure the heartbeat of one person being registered in the other person's brainwaves.[10] (Fig. F) By learning to create internal entrainment and coherence through the FREEZE-FRAME process, you radiate a much more harmonious signal to your environment and the people around you.

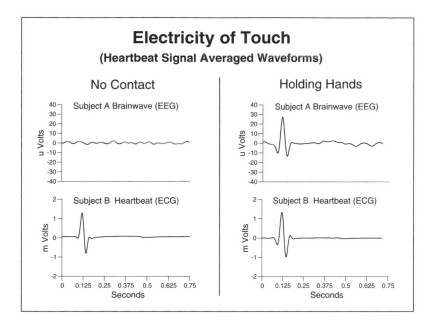

Figure F. Electricity of Touch
Signal averaging techniques were used to show that when two individuals touch, one person's electrocardiogram (ECG—heartbeat) signal is registered in the other person's electroencephalogram (EEG—brainwave) and elsewhere on the person's body.

Beyond 2000—Freeze-Framing in Action

In late 1993, a videotape crew from the television program *Beyond 2000* came to the Institute's research facility to do a feature on the music *Heart Zones*, which I designed scientifically to help people achieve increased mental and emotional balance and renewed vitality. The crew wanted to understand how the music was created, how to use it to get better results with FREEZE-FRAME and how we were able to prove its effectiveness in our laboratory research.

The host for the show decided to open the segment by being hooked up to all the physiological testing equipment in the lab—heart rate, ECG, EEG (brainwaves), blood pressure, respiration and more. Computers tracked all his physiological responses as he was videotaped. Unfortunately, he stumbled over his opening lines several times, forcing repeated "takes" and he became increasingly tense and nervous. The computers showed the results of his mounting tension. His blood pressure and heart rate had shot up to extremely high levels. The scientist monitoring the host's physiological responses suggested he try the FREEZE-FRAME technique he had learned earlier. As you can see in Figure G, within seconds his heart rate and blood pressure returned to normal and his respiration regained a smooth, even pattern. He then delivered his lines perfectly. The host and crew were delighted that they had real-time verification of FREEZE-FRAME's effectiveness captured on videotape.

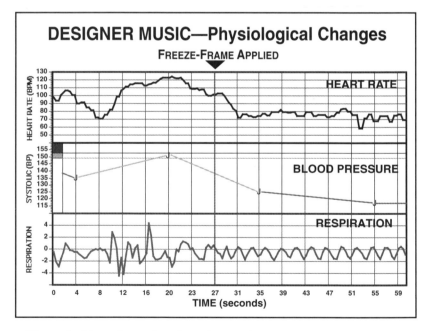

Figure G. Chart shows the effect of *Heart Zones* and FREEZE-FRAME on an individual with little prior training. The individual was the host of the TV show *Beyond 2000* featured on the Discovery Channel.

Heart Hormones and the Immune System

Scientists are proving that repeated episodes of anger and frustration cause nervous system imbalances that are detrimental not only to the heart, but to the brain and the hormonal and immune systems. Have you ever had an argument with someone you loved and, the next day, replayed the situation over and over in your mind, cranking up negative emotions from the day before that made you feel terrible? Even recalling an upsetting episode can produce imbalances and stress. As mentioned earlier, the stress reaction creates specific hormonal imbalances and that these same hormonal imbalances have been shown to damage brain cells. They may even lead to Alzheimer's disease.[11] It doesn't have to be that way once you understand what you are doing to yourself and how you can change it.

A study conducted at the HeartMath Research Center recently demonstrated that a group of normal, healthy people were able to increase the amount of the hormone DHEA available to the cells by up to 100% while decreasing their cortisol levels by 23%.[12] DHEA is a very important hormone and is often referred to as the "anti-aging" hormone while cortisol is called the "stress hormone" because it is well known to increase when you are experiencing stress or feeling anxiety, helplessness or withdrawal. Cortisol is also the hormone that can damage the brain cells when its levels are kept too high from constant stress or worry. In the study, the increase in DHEA was significantly related to the subjects' increasing their feeling of warmheartedness; the reduction in cortisol was related to their reductions in stress levels after practicing a HeartMath tool[13] and listening to the music I wrote to facilitate the process. This stress-reducing music has been shown in other research studies to help boost immunity,[14] reduce tension and improve mental clarity.[15] (Figure H)

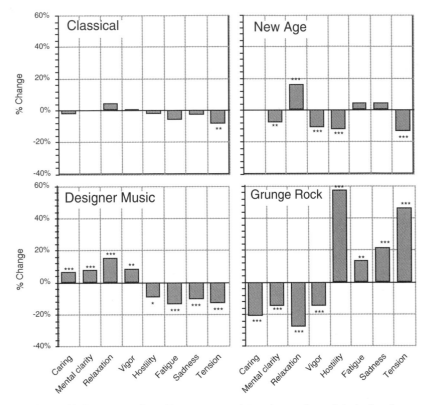

Figure H. Compares the effects on mood, tension and mental clarity of listening to designer music (*Speed of Balance*) compared to three other music genres (classical, new age and grunge rock). Shows percentage change in mood, tension and mental clarity for each category of music. *Speed of Balance* produced significant increases in all positive scales: caring, relaxation, mental clarity and vigor. Significant decreases were produced in all negative scales: hostility, fatigue, sadness and tension.

The Immune System's First Line of Defense

IgA (immunoglobulin A) is an immune system antibody and one of the body's first lines of defense against colds, flu and infections of the respiratory and urinary tracts. IgA is found in our saliva, lungs, digestive and urinary systems. In a group study (twenty individuals) comparing the effects of anger versus care and compassion on average IgA levels, it was found that one five-minute episode of mentally and emotionally recalling an experience of anger caused an immediate short-term rise in IgA, followed by a depletion that was so severe it took the body more than six hours to restore normal production of IgA (see Figure I). What this study showed is that even a single episode of recalling an experience of anger and frustration can depress your immune system for almost an entire day.[16]

Figure I.

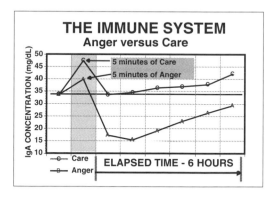

Figure I. This graph shows the impact of one 5-minute episode of recalled anger on the immune antibody IgA over a six-hour period. The initial slight increase in IgA was followed by a dramatic drop which persisted for six hours. When the subjects used the FREEZE-FRAME technique and focused on feeling sincere care for five minutes, there was a significant increase in IgA, which returned to baseline an hour later and then slowly increased throughout the rest of the day.

What are most people's days like? You wake up anxious because you didn't sleep well; you get frustrated with a co-worker who forgot to give you an important report; somebody gives you a strange look at the coffee machine and you feel a surge of irritation. Then you find 15 voicemail messages that you're late responding to—it's a cascading series of events of anxiety, frustration and anger. The cumulative results of seemingly insignificant frustrations and anxieties have been shown to be even more detrimental to the immune system than the occasional large blowout of anger.[17] Is it any wonder that health care costs are so high, eating up a huge percentage of corporate profits and expected to get worse?

This same IgA study also showed that one five-minute episode of mentally and emotionally experiencing the emotions of care and compassion caused a much larger, immediate rise in IgA—an average of 34%—followed by a return to normal (baseline).[16] However, the IgA levels then gradually climbed above baseline throughout the next six hours. Learning to manage the moment and increase the ratio of your positive attitudes and feelings can improve your quality of life and well-being.

Other studies also show that feelings of happiness and joy increase white blood cell counts needed for healing[18] and defend against invading pathogens, including cancer and virus-infected cells.

FREEZE-FRAME with HIV-positive/AIDS patients

In a study using FREEZE-FRAME with HIV-positive and AIDS patients, researchers found dramatic improvements in anxiety levels and physical symptoms. Using the STAI (State Trait Anxiety Inventory) to measure psychological changes, participants who practiced FREEZE-FRAME for six months reduced their level of despair, anger, fear and guilt. At the beginning of the study, most of the participants had very high levels of anxiety. This was quite understandable considering the condition of their health and the general prognosis for people diagnosed HIV-positive. By the end of the six-month study, average anxiety levels had dropped by 20%, almost to that of the average healthy person, in spite of the fact that they still had a virus that is feared by society and could supposedly kill them at any time.[19] They also reported more balance and harmonious flow throughout the day. More things seemed to go their way and they were able to increase the percentage of good days and get more done.

Affiliative Motive

Another psychological measure is, the "affiliative motive." Affiliation is a social motive characterized by the desire to establish warm and caring relationships with others. People with strong affiliative motive tend to be loving and caring individuals. It has been shown that loving and caring people have decreased levels of stress hormones, and higher IgA levels during times of stress than non-affiliative individuals.[20] They get sick less often and are less vulnerable to disease.[21] Loving and caring people also have increased norepinephrine, a chemical released from the nerves that has a wide variety of functions in balancing the nervous systems.[22] Studies have shown that even if you aren't naturally affiliative, self-induced feelings of warmth and care towards others also increase IgA levels,[23] resulting in an enhanced immune system.

Easy Access

The FREEZE-FRAME technology focuses your attention in the area around the heart (where people subjectively feel love, care and appreciation). These feelings have been shown to help balance the nervous systems.[7] When you FREEZE-FRAME, the heart rhythms become smooth and coherent and the signals that the heart sends to the brain through the nervous system affect the perceptual centers in the brain. This helps to give you a more balanced perspective of any situation.

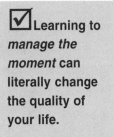
☑ Learning to *manage the moment* can literally change the quality of your life.

FREEZE-FRAME is a technology that gives you the conscious ability to self-manage your reactions, gain clarity and have more quality, fun and well-being in the moment. You gain the power to make better choices and decisions and not be victimized by your reactions to people, places and situations. Just as the detrimental effects of stress are cumulative, so are the beneficial effects of FREEZE-FRAME. Practice leads to increased mental and emotional buoyancy, cardiovascular efficiency and improved quality of life. Here's how it works inside our body:

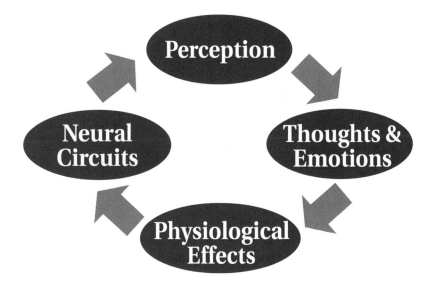

The Cycle of Perception— Reprogramming Neural Circuitry

Your perceptions underlie how you think and feel about the person or issue that you are dealing with. The resulting thoughts and emotions, but especially the emotions, cause numerous physiological changes in the body. These changes can be measured in the nervous system, hormonal system, heart and blood pressure. These changes, in turn, feed back and affect what is called the neural circuitry of the brain. The state of your neural circuitry, in turn, affects your perception. Your neural circuitry consists of neural pathways in the brain and body, pathways that are developed and reinforced to the degree that we use them. Whether you "learn" a healthy response or a stressful reaction, you are "hard-wiring" this pattern into your system through repetition.

Here's an illustration of how the cycle works. If you get frustrated because traffic was unusually heavy on the way to work, that feeling causes the sympathetic nervous system to increase your heart rate and instruct the adrenal glands to secrete adrenaline and other hormones into the blood stream. These

"If you change your perception, you change the experience of your body and your world."

Deepak Chopra, M.D.

45

changes then affect the neural circuits in the brain. You are then more sensitive to the next stressful situation and more likely to have a negative reaction. If you repeat this pattern, the neural pathways in the brain are reinforced and your emotional response becomes automatic so that you can get stuck in repeating, inefficient thought loops such as worry and anxiety. This then leads to a depletion of your energy and clouds your judgment. FREEZE-FRAME allows you to break the cycle, and with practice you can begin to retrain and reprogram the neural circuitry so that you are not the victim of your own thought loops and inappropriate self-defeating emotional reactions, but can build new intelligence into your system.

Promoting Physical Health and Vitality

Chapter 4

CHAPTER HIGHLIGHTS

* Relieving Illness
* Implications for Health
* Staying Youthful
* Enhancing Your Sports Edge

"These techniques have made an amazing difference to team morale. Before trying it, 46% said they often felt exhausted; after the training, this figure fell to 9%. Some staff members even said they felt kinder." [1]

Carol Mortimer, Director of Healthcare, Hewlett-Packard, (U.K.)

As you read in the previous chapter, FREEZE-FRAME has been shown to calm and smooth the heart rhythms, boost the immune system and reduce symptoms of stress. For many, this could mean a general improvement in health and an intelligent preventative against more serious situations. But for those who are already dealing with chronic health conditions, practicing FREEZE-FRAME can mean the difference between leading a normal healthy life—or not.

Checklist for Physical Stress

Which of these physical stresses apply to you?

❑ Frequent aches or pains (headaches, backaches, stomach problems, heartburn, others)

❑ Too many colds, congestion or respiratory ailments that last longer than you'd like

❑ Frequent fatigue or feeling run down

❑ Chronic or major illness

❑ Accident prone

Following are a couple of case studies that illustrate the importance of having healthy, coherent heart rhythms. They also show the value of being able to control your emotional reactions, and therefore the sequence of biological events that determine your health.

Heart Arrhythmia

Two years before Patricia came to HeartMath, her heart was beating 700 extra beats per hour. On betablockers, valium and aspirin daily, her hair was falling out, she had stomach aches, headaches and was told she was at risk of sudden death. During this time she survived a near-fatal ventricular tachycardia episode (during which the heart beats at very high speeds for extended periods of time), had surgery four times and had to take an extended sick leave from her high-level job at a global computer company.

"I was the type of person who was trying to be the perfect mother, the perfect wife, the perfect employee. I used to sleep four hours a night because there was so much to do. I thrived on it. I was so used to that adrenaline rush, that I didn't know what it was like not to have it."

Patricia attended a HeartMath seminar in the fall of 1995 and immediately began to practice FREEZE-FRAME on a regular basis. "After my weekend at HeartMath, whenever that adrenaline would start to rush again, I could stop the trigger. The first day back to work, I got up eight times and went to the ladies room, shut myself in and closed my eyes. That's when I did the FREEZE-FRAME. Now, I don't need to close my eyes and can pull myself back into balance without going anywhere."

Her colleagues immediately noticed a difference—less stress and tension and more ease, even during particularly hectic work periods. Her cardiologist and her specialists at Stanford University were particularly impressed.

Within a few weeks she was off of valium; within 5 months the betablocker that controls her arrhythmia was decreased by half; within nine months she had a normal 24-hour ECG recording. There have been no further episodes of ventricular tachycardia or further surgery. There were no lifestyle, dietary or exercise changes; therefore, Patricia attributes these profound improvements to FREEZE-FRAME. Nearly three years later, Patricia has her life back and now feels "calm and absolutely incredible."

Joseph Chilton Pearce, author of *Magical Child* and *Evolution's End*, has become a friend and regular visitor at HeartMath since his dramatic health turnaround. "I suffered from severe arrhythmia, atrial fibrillation and tachycardia, a life-threatening condition. My heart would stop beating for 4 to 5 beats, then come back with a pound on my chest and a heart rate of 160 beats per minute. Doctors had me on betablockers and other medications. Then I was introduced to HeartMath. Within two weeks of practicing the HeartMath tools [FREEZE-FRAME] my condition improved dramatically and I was able to stop taking the betablockers. I've had only one or two episodes since and have lived medication-free for the past three years. I am doing all I can to spread the word about HeartMath."

It's amazing how much healing and regenerative power the human system has when body, mind and emotions are in sync rather than fighting each other. As research has proven, when your unmanaged emotions fuel negative thought patterns, you pay a price in accelerated aging, weakened immune system and impaired cardiovascular function. Letting excessive negative emotion blow through your system is like having a big hole blow right through your balloon of energy. Everything can be drained out of you in a matter of moments. It can take hours, days, even weeks to recover. Some people suffer this so frequently, they never "recover." They never experience the kind of vitality that comes with emotional balance.

Chronic Fatigue Syndrome

When fatigue persists for at least six months and other symptoms develop, it is called chronic fatigue. In another research study conducted by HeartMath Research Center, people with chronic fatigue were found to have low autonomic nervous system (ANS) function.

Rollin McCraty, IHM's research director, reports: "What we now believe is that in many, but not all, cases of fatigue and chronic fatigue, the extra wear and tear from stress placed on the autonomic nervous system and the glands and organs they control, depletes the nervous system.

"This manifests as low heart rate variability, a sign of increased aging. Once this happens it is hard to recover unless the stress cycle is broken and steps are taken to help the nervous system recover.

"We have seen a number of people with fatigue recover in a relatively short time by sincerely using the FREEZE-FRAME and Heart Lock-In®* technologies. FREEZE-FRAME helps break the stress cycle and Heart Lock-In helps retrain the nervous system by locking in the more harmonious and coherent patterns which allow it to regenerate and recover.

"IHM has conducted a number of research studies in large corporations. In many of these studies we find high levels of fatigue and burnout among the employees. We also see high levels of sleeplessness, tension and other physical symptoms of stress. After practicing the tools we see significant reductions in fatigue and the other stress symptoms in the people."

Patrick Jacobs, a nuclear and electronic computing engineer, shares the story of his struggle with chronic fatigue and how recognizing and shifting in the moment can improve even chronic conditions.

"After a trip to Mexico in 1984, I returned with a variety of symptoms beginning a downward spiral leading to collapse in the fall of 1986. My energy was gone. I was unable to think, unable to get out of bed—only waking for about an hour a day, and during that hour sometimes able to only open my eyes. It was 4 months before I could walk to the mailbox. That chore used to take me 5 minutes. Now it took at least half an hour.

"To this day, there is still no identified cause for chronic fatigue syndrome, so the medical community treats the symptoms. If you can't sleep, they give you something to help you sleep better. If you have pain or are depressed, they give you medications for those problems.

*Heart Lock-In is another technique taught at HeartMath seminars and in the *HeartMath Discovery Program*.

"My next 10 years were marked by gradual progress to very fragile plateaus. I was learning to operate in a very reduced way. Yet, it was a delicate balancing act—I had no idea when the next wave of depletion would knock me off my feet. Not knowing if this was ever going to be over was extremely frustrating.

"During recovery from my last major relapse in the fall of 1994, I recognized something major was missing from my strategy but I didn't have a clue what that was. In the spring of 1995, I came upon an article on the research of the Institute of HeartMath.

"I began learning the HeartMath techniques [FREEZE-FRAME] for managing thoughts and emotions and bringing the autonomic nervous system into balance—first with the books and tapes, then a weekend retreat. I'm using the techniques on a very regular basis, and catching the first signs of the illness and shifting out of it before going down. The changes have been miraculous!

"With chronic fatigue, you can't really plan your life, even a couple of days ahead. Using HeartMath, I am experiencing the increased energy and mental function I've needed to really reenter life in a stable way. Now I've gotten to the point where I can ask the question, what do I want to do with the rest of my life? This is a very exciting place to be. For the first time in my life it seems like all my resources are aligning, providing hope and a deeper sense of peace."

These are just a few of the many documented stories we have received from people who have improved their health by using the FREEZE-FRAME technique. FREEZE-FRAME has also been shown to improve physical conditions such as hypertension, migraine headaches, general fatigue, tension, rapid heartbeats, body aches, indigestion and sleep disorders. Since the technique has been shown to improve autonomic nervous system balance, it can be useful for conditions associated with autonomic imbalance, such as arrythmia, hypertension, coronary artery disease, mitral valve prolapse, depression, irritable bowel, asthma, diabetes, hypoglycemia and fibromyalgia.

If you are faced with a health challenge, feel run down or have an annoying ache or pain, try Freeze-Framing. (This is not instead of taking medication that might be appropriate, but as an add-on.) Let the body quiet down for a few moments while you calm the mind and emotions. Frequently, the annoyance you feel when the physical body is hurting or sick only adds to the discomfort and lengthens the healing process. By using FREEZE-FRAME on a regular basis, you boost your immune system and maintain a coherent, healthy inner environment so that your body can save energy and remain youthful and strong.

Staying Flexible and Youthful

We all would love to find the fountain of youth. But to come upon a big waterfall labeled "Drink here; you've found it!" might not happen. Let's take a subtler look at what youth really means on the inside.

Everyone knows how refreshing a child's energy can be. Children have a certain liquid flexibility that "goes with the flow." They play with all their hearts and if they fall down and scrape their knee, once the bandage is on, they're usually back into the swing of things fast. To find an adult with these same qualities is not so easy. What happened to us? Where did it go? Did our spirits age too? That's what a fountain would be good for—to fill us back up with childlike qualities of enthusiasm, flexibility and the zest for adventure no matter how difficult your life experience has been.

Slowing the Aging Process

Do you feel age setting in? Aging is a part of life. But to age naturally, with a childlike heart, can keep the sparkle, spontaneity and adventure in your life.

To age mentally and emotionally denotes a loss of flexibility and a loss of the ability to adapt. You become a person who doesn't like to do anything you don't usually do—and nobody can change your mind. You become "set in stone." You've lost the childlike feeling that life's an adventure, with new events to experience and enjoy.

From a scientific perspective, aging happens when your cells lose flexibility and the ability to adapt. You become crystallized in certain habits and attitudes that are harder and harder to change. But it's being proven in the lab that the positive hormones you create within your own system with positive feelings do more for your regeneration than you might know.

Remember, FREEZE-FRAME is a one-minute technique. It's like a Swiss Army knife—a convenient tool to use anywhere. What if you have an opportunity to go on a camping trip with friends, but have to give up your usual routine for a few days in order to get ready? After all, there are bags to pack, supplies to gather, plants to water, pets to feed. What a hassle! The further you explore it, it's really too much trouble. It just wouldn't be worth it.

If you are "set in your ways," find yourself "stuck on principle" and are unable to make a flexible decision, FREEZE-FRAME. Shift your thoughts away from knowing what you know about yourself. Focus your attention in your heart and go to neutral. Hold that for a moment or two. Then ask yourself—without the "I don't want to's" or the "I think I should's" interfering—what would be the most rewarding thing to do?

Recall what it feels like to be with friends, laughing, having fun and going on adventures. If that camping trip still doesn't feel right for you, you have at least given it a fair shot. Take that moment and find clarity on what you really want to do, beneath the usual mind resistances and thoughts like, "It's just not convenient." This way, after the car pulls out and the friends are off to play, you won't have any second thoughts or regret your choice. So much stress is created by people wishing they'd made different decisions in life. As you learn to make peace with life as it is, you develop more power to change it for the better.

A New Lease on Life

Hobart Johnson was born with cerebral palsy. In 1990 he had a stroke due to stress in his job as a marketing executive for a software firm. In the months following the stroke his blood pressure fluctuated up to the 200/100 range. His disability forced this dynamic Stanford Business School graduate into an early retirement.

The beginning of 1994 marked his first visit to the Institute of HeartMath. "At that time," he recalls, "people in my life gave me six months to live. I had a deteriorating condition, high blood pressure, I was unable to walk without a cane and had basically lost interest in life due to the progressive nature of the condition."

After being immersed in the HeartMath process for four years, practicing FREEZE-FRAME at every opportunity during the day, he says,

"It just keeps getting better. My blood pressure is now 150/70, my heart and circulation are normal. I have reentered the workplace part time. I am much calmer and happier with life. I'm told I look 10 years younger than my 67 years, and I feel it too. I am alive again and thoroughly appreciate the new world in which I find myself."

I'm not saying FREEZE-FRAME is intended to be the fountain of youth, a new religion or new philosophy. People have to work out their own beliefs about life within themselves. However, this tool can often "save your tail" while you try to work all that out for yourself. It's a simple, scientific approach to your own health and well-being. Don't let the simplicity throw you. Because Freeze-Framing was so simple, we went through painstaking experiments in the lab to prove or disprove its effectiveness. It's the very simplicity of FREEZE-FRAME that's creating all the testimonies of excitement.

Enhancing Your Sports Edge

Playing sports can be one of your most fun and regenerating activities, but sports is also a major source of stress for many. For example, a 1994 survey of golfers in Japan revealed that pressure to perform well at golf is causing an alarming number of heart attacks. Most people who enjoy sports want to improve their health—not lose it—while they sharpen their game.

If you're a sports enthusiast, you may have lofty expectations of your own performance. Competition can breed tremendous pressure, especially if self-image, money or a prize is involved. People react to this pressure by getting tense at exactly the time they need mental and physical flexibility. The outcome can be mental and physical under-performance known as "choking in the clutch." Great players have the ability to stay loose and make the great play. FREEZE-FRAME technology has been proven to help people stay loose under pressure while enhancing their passion for achievement.

Increasingly, people are waking up to the importance of getting their mind and emotions entrained for sustained success. Entrainment occurs when your heart rhythms are harmonious, your parasympathetic and sympathetic nervous systems are in balance, and your mind and emotions feel in sync. All systems are in tune.

Pete Sampras, consistently the number one-ranked tennis player in the world for several years, has become famous for his focused, even-keeled nature during competition. He doesn't get overly excited when he makes a great shot nor overly disturbed when he blows a shot. He has a sense of humor that helps him stay balanced without suppressing his emotions. Recently, one of the world's top ranked players of the '80s and winner of several Grand Slams stated that if he had managed his emotions better during his career, he would have won more matches. The FREEZE-FRAME technique is an excellent way to increase your leverage in any sport without sacrificing your fun or your health.

Finding the Groove—A Golf Note

As you read in Chapter 3, when you practice FREEZE-FRAME, the two branches of the autonomic nervous system become more balanced and efficient. In addition the heart rate variability pattern becomes smooth and even. The information the heart sends via the nervous system to the brain facilitates motor skills, coordination, reaction speeds, mental clarity and focus. A balanced nervous system insures a higher ratio of smooth and fluid mind/body coherence, where you experience the "flow."

Incoherence in the nervous system, for a golfer, can result in poor performance, including the "yips"—a slight jerk or twitch most noticeable while putting. Using FREEZE-FRAME can enhance the performance of both the individual and the team in any sport, and makes the game much more enjoyable.

Lynn Marriott is a PGA and LPGA Class A professional golfer and Director of Golf Education at Arizona State University Karsten Golf Course. Lynn explains why more pros are using FREEZE-FRAME to improve their golf game. "At the elite level, poor performance is often a result of indecision. These players all have the technical skill, so that's not what determines the winner. What's critical is the ability to make a clear decision about the shot, to be able to sort through all the details and stressors about the course and each particular shot. When a player is grounded and trusts their intuition about the shot, there is no indecision. Using FREEZE-FRAME to shift from your head to your heart throughout your game increases the clarity about your golf shot.

"For instance, use FREEZE-FRAME in your pre-shot routine, just before your last look at the target. You get grounded, center in the heart, and the feeling comes, 'yes, go.' Sometimes you stand over a putt and you know the ball is going in—other times you stand over a putt and can't access that same confidence and clarity. FREEZE-FRAME helps you access your 'go' signals more easily."

Lynn's friend and colleague, Pia Nilsson, is head coach for the Swedish Golf Federation and the European Solheim Cup Captain. Pia attended a HeartMath training and now uses FREEZE-FRAME both in her own game and in her coaching. In her new book, *Be Your Own Best Coach* Pia talks about FREEZE-

FRAME and says, "One of the future keys to better golf is to literally play from the heart."

Better than Ever

D ennis Kelly, author of *Six Steps to the Fountain of Youth* writes about how a simple shift in perspective can affect vitality.

"In my thirties, I entered tournaments and won awards in the martial arts, but my life had taken a turn for the worst. Drastic financial problems and having my very ill parents come to live with me had left me devoid of hope and filled with bitterness. I abandoned my passion and retired from sports altogether.

"Then one day a friend introduced me to FREEZE-FRAME. I recognized that it was in tune with the martial arts centering techniques I'd practiced for years, but it went several steps further! The master trainers had always spoken about the heart but not in the clear how-to-get-there-and-use-it kind of way.

"After practicing the techniques, my whole attitude changed. I realized that there is no reason to let life's obstacles prevent me from doing the things I loved. I wouldn't let it get me down.

"In January, 1997, I came out of retirement and entered competition again. I'm pleased to say that, at 59, I'm the oldest man ever to win a world championship in the sparring division with NASKA (North American Sport Karate Association.)

"The curious thing is that, when I was 20 years younger, the competition was far less intense. I won awards then, but I was mainly fighting with amateurs. Nowadays, pros and masters can compete in the 40+ division. It was a much more difficult challenge to win—yet, with the focus I gained from this technique, my performance was far better at 59 years old than it had been in my '30s!!"

People who watch sports also experience stress. Some get so over-identified when their team loses, they remain upset for days and manufacture stress-producing hormones the whole time. Using FREEZE-FRAME presents a chance for the heart to tell the mind to release and let go because a lost game is not going to undo itself. Repetitive over-identity with losing induces stress on the heart and immune system, often resulting in physical ailments.

Freeze-Framing isn't intended to take the excitement and drama out of watching or playing sports. It's designed to give you the focus and flexibility to enhance your performance, so you can enjoy the stress-free fun of the sport, where your body, mind and emotions are in sync. By maintaining the poise of *it's only a game*, if the outcome isn't to your liking, you won't take it out on your family, coworkers or your immune system.

Managing Your Emotions

Chapter 5

CHAPTER HIGHLIGHTS

- **About Emotions**
- **Using FREEZE-FRAME with Fear and Anxiety**
- **Overcoming Depression**

When emotions are brought back to balance, your mind has a chance to achieve clear common sense.

People live for the moments when their hearts come alive. That doesn't just mean at holiday time, extra special events or peak moments. FREEZE-FRAME is especially designed to help you activate positive feelings in your heart *at will*. Many people feel so unloved or unliked they find it hard to feel love, especially for themselves. Millions suffer from mood swings—feeling great one minute and terrible the next. Mood-altering drugs are in great demand because people simply want to feel better more of the time.

Your most productive drugs are those within your own endocrine system. You feel alive and have additional energy and vitality when your hormonal flow is optimized. You influence this flow more than you may realize by how much you manage your mental and emotional perceptions and reactions. You are your own pharmacist. Learning to put your emotions in balance helps you access the inner prescription that accomplishes the best overall health.

Emotions are neutral. Depending on the perception that triggers the emotion, they can either provide warmth, vibrancy and clarity to your experience, or be like a dark cloud, making it difficult to see solutions. FREEZE-FRAME will help you calm and balance your emotions so they won't keep rampaging through your mind.

I'm not trying to imply that your emotions are a negative force in the human system or that you should try to suppress them. I am saying that you'll save energy when you learn to first neutralize their intent before you engage them. When the heat of the emotions is turned down, the mind can see more options and more solutions.

When the emotions are managed, not suppressed, they can be used to add more fun, texture and quality to life. They are like free fuel for your system; if left unmanaged, they can be highly flammable. As you find emotional maturity, through balance between your heart and your head, your emotions turn into creative passion and become a tremendous asset. Creatively directing that focused passion is fun. To turn emotional deficits into rewarding assets, we first need to recognize emotional stress.

P sychologist Pam Aasen, Ph.D., has been recommending FREEZE-FRAME to her patients with great success. She says,

"People with a history of trauma or chronic stress may develop a high tolerance for stress and can be unaware of day-to-day stress and its impact on physical, mental and emotional well-being."

She encourages her patients with chronic stress to practice FREEZE-FRAME regularly so they can begin to recognize stressors. "With practice, the positive state of well-being experienced from regular use of this heart power tool can help you establish a baseline for healthy stress awareness. It will start to become uncomfortable to experience stress when you know there is a positive alternative that you can use whenever you start to feel uneasy. This way, you can start to develop a healthy intolerance for stress discomfort."

Venting Your Emotions

How many times have you heard someone say, "It felt good to get angry and tell that S.O.B. off." It can feel good in the moment to get your emotions out. Emotional outbursts are tricky. Getting them out is usually better than holding them in. The problem is that emotional outbursts often come with a price tag of additional stress and another mess to clean up later.

Emotional Checklist

Which of these emotional stresses apply to you?

❑ **Irritation**

❑ **Feeling unloved or unliked**

❑ **Frustration**

❑ **Frequent hurt feelings**

❑ **Anger**

❑ **Afraid of losing control**

❑ **Anxiety**

❑ **Fears or phobias**

❑ **Moodiness**

❑ **Depression**

Often times the person you've dumped on doesn't remember your message; they just remember the onslaught. Your approach hasn't solved the problem. You've probably just added to it. As you learn to FREEZE-FRAME highly-charged emotions, you also learn to communicate directly to people without the extra voltage that can cause them to be defensive, while frying your nerves and draining your energy bank.

Dr. Joseph McCaffrey, a general and vascular surgeon at an upstate New York hospital, discovered the value-added benefits of Freeze-Framing to avoid an otherwise fully-justified emotional outburst.

"I recently had a high-risk patient scheduled for surgery on a gall bladder. He was all prepped in the holding area and waiting to be taken in for the operation. His anesthesiologist had approved him for surgery. But the anesthesiologist in the Operating Room (OR) insisted the patient needed another cardiac workup, which meant we'd have to cancel the surgery. After discussion, I reluctantly agreed, canceled the surgery, explained the situation to Bill and his family and consulted the cardiologist. The cardiologist saw Bill later that night and cleared him for surgery.

"The next day was Friday. I had a 4 hour vascular operation scheduled and added Bill to follow. It turned out to be the first hot day of the season. The air conditioning hadn't kicked in yet. It was over 80° in the OR!

"Hot and exhausted at 2:00 PM, I finished one operation and headed for the next when I learned the OR anesthesiologist had canceled again! I was stewing. Bill's anesthesiologist was stewing too. He took it as a professional affront. In typical form, I started in on the OR guy: 'Who do you think you are? How could you presume...Not even your patient —' I got about two sentences in and I stopped. I knew I could win, but I thought, 'This isn't great. I know where this goes. Even if I win the battle, it will cost me. It'll be hard to work with this guy for awhile and the tension will reverberate throughout the entire department. It isn't worth it.'

"I did a FREEZE-FRAME on the spot which shifted my perspective immediately. I realized that none of these doctors was trying to be lazy. We all just wanted the best thing for the patient. I could appreciate that basically it was a reasonable difference of professional opinion, and we had a bunch of well-intended, dedicated people. As I shifted the tone of the conversation, the others followed suit. We started speaking to each other respectfully, as colleagues, instead of hostile opponents.

"Over the next few days, we experienced a creative collaboration that would never have happened had I followed my initial reaction. We identified the problem areas that had emerged and crafted some changes to the hospital policy to insure the problems didn't reoccur. Thanks to FREEZE-FRAME, it was a dynamic, creative and amazingly productive session."

Using FREEZE-FRAME for Fear and Anxiety

Many people live in fear: fear of rejection, fear of loss, fear of being hurt, fear of the future, fear of change—the list of phobias is long. While it is not my intention in this book to address the emotion of fear in great detail, I know that many fears can be lessened through engaging the power of your heart to help calm fear reactions and gain more objectivity. For instance, if you are especially prone to anxiety, it is a good idea to begin building your FREEZE-FRAME muscle before an anxiety-producing situation happens. You do this by simply finding something or someone to appreciate several times a day, though you may feel you don't need to.

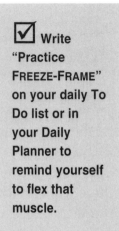

☑ Write "Practice FREEZE-FRAME" on your daily To Do list or in your Daily Planner to remind yourself to flex that muscle.

Psychiatrist Jeffrey Stevens, M.D., director of an Idaho hospital pain and anxiety clinic, is launching a FREEZE-FRAME research project to reduce the stress on the psychiatric staff and increase the quality of patient care. Dr. Stevens says, "I've taught many patients the basic FREEZE-FRAME technique with very good success, especially people with anxiety problems. In one case, an extremely nervous patient I've seen for years, who never responded to multiple psychological and pharmacological interventions did so well with FREEZE-FRAME that at first she didn't recognize herself, she was so used to being nervous all the time. She was just delighted.

I've had wonderful results using FREEZE-FRAME with anxieties, phobias and panic. I have not seen an obvious group of people that can't do it; though persons who have extreme difficulty taking responsibility for their thoughts and feelings can be challenging."

Financial Anxiety

Issues like money can trigger feelings of anxiety in most people. While it may not immobilize you, it can still eat away at your peace and happiness.

One San Francisco single mother learned to recognize and deal with her financial anxiety in a healthy way. "Since becoming a single mother 7 years ago and handling my finances for the first time, I had noticed an ever-increasing, palpable dread over loss of security and fear of spending too impulsively, even though I had a very secure job and enough money to support my family. I needed to find some way to help me feel calm in the crazy moments of my day-to-day living as a teacher and parent, when all the little things begin to grow way out of proportion. The very first time I did a FREEZE-FRAME, I asked myself about the consuming fears I had around money.

"My FREEZE-FRAME question was, 'How can I overcome my anxiety around money?' I had not expected the oddball answer that came out of left field—'give more!'— not at all something my normal thinking would have produced. I began to act on it and the effect on my life has been profound. I realized that the emotion of anxiety came from the thought that money was scarce. So I began reversing to an abundance mindset—feeling secure—and increasing my giving in all manner of ways. Not just money, but my time, skill, caring, attention and affection. Not only has the fear been dramatically reduced, but new fulfilling opportunities have come my way.

"Now, when I feel the clutches of worry, I can just park my fears and say, 'see ya' later' instead of going into an energy tailspin of irritability and depression the way I used to do. Shifting into 'neutral' is the antidote to worry. FREEZE-FRAME and neutral are the most instantly accessible and reliable tools for problem solving and de-stressing I've ever used. I can trust them to be there whenever I need them."

Public Speaking Anxiety

It is said that the biggest fear people have—next to dying—is speaking in public. It's better to find a place of neutral, relaxing the knot in your stomach or the quiver in your voice, so you're no longer paralyzed by your fear. With practice, the technique will activate positive feelings and perspectives that can actually release the fear. We hear many stories of how people use FREEZE-FRAME to overcome their fear of speaking in public.

A dramatic example comes from a former assistant police chief of San Jose, California. "During my 30-year career, I've been required to make many speeches and I've also taught at the college level for seven years. I've developed an ability to speak in front of a classroom of fifty without any problem.

"When I became Assistant Chief, I was asked to speak in front of a packed convention hall of 500 police officers and their families for a promotional ceremony.

"It was really a shock when I walked in there. I was well-prepared because preparation is supposed to reduce anxiety, but I got tremendously anxious. I became very warm and started to perspire. I said to myself, 'This is not me.' I'm normally under control so much better than that. I have negotiated hostage situations but at that moment I would rather have been negotiating a hostage release than making that speech. So I Freeze-Framed and an unbelievable calm came over me just before I had to begin. I spoke from the heart and really didn't look over my notes. It went over beautifully. Afterwards, I received several comments from people who said it had been the best speech they had ever heard during a promotional ceremony. One woman even came up to me saying it was the first time she had wanted to cry at one of these ceremonies."

> I Freeze-Framed and an unbelievable calm came over me before I had to begin.

68

Tips on Practicing FREEZE-FRAME for Anxiety

—From Dr. Pam Aasen

☑ Practice FREEZE-FRAME when you are not anxious so you can develop a positive association with the tools and *Heart Zones* music*. If you practice FREEZE-FRAME only when you are experiencing anxiety or having a panic attack, you may begin to associate FREEZE-FRAME with anxiety and distress rather than relief and comfort.

☑ Establish a list of 8-10 memories or experiences which are calming and comforting to you. Practice FREEZE-FRAME with each of these positive experiences to build the strength of these calming and comforting memories so when you feel anxious and stressed, you can easily access these feeling memories and be comforted by them.

☑ If your mind tends to wander to the future and antici-pate negative outcomes, gently return your attention to the present and refocus on your heart. Try to feel your "soft heart" or the warmth in the center of your chest. Take a deep, slow "heart breath" to refocus on the present. Re-member, ruminating and anticipation keep you depressed and anxious by taking you out of the heart and into negative thought loops in your mind.

*Publisher's note: *Heart Zones'* (Doc Childre's instrumental music re-cording) ability to enhance the beneficial effects of positive emotional states on autonomic and immune function has been documented in *Stress Medicine* (Vol 12:167-175).

Tips...

☑ As stress develops, you can use FREEZE-FRAME to avoid creating an "anxiety mountain" out of a "stress mole-hill." Molehills may be a challenge but most of us can manage the short-term discomfort of a molehill. Mountains, however, seem overwhelming and we are all inclined to avoid the mountains that overwhelm us.

☑ If you follow the guidance of your FREEZE-FRAME heart insights, you can minimize anxiety and the overwhelming feelings that drain your energy while building confidence in your own heart power. Action on the problems will minimize future anxiety and stress. One of the major advantages of using FREEZE-FRAME for anxiety is that when you do the technique, you experience entrainment which makes it much easier to act on the problem. Life becomes easier.

Overcoming Depression

Depression is an emotional distress call suffered by millions. A woman with chronic depression had been seeing a psychiatrist, taking lithium for over a year, but wasn't improving. Her husband and two young children were distraught that they were unable to help. After reading one of our books, *The Hidden Power of the Heart*, she attended a Heart Empowerment® training and had a private consultation with a HeartMath trainer. The trainer noticed the woman was constantly voicing how terrible a person she was, invariably putting herself down. She asked the woman to practice Freeze-Framing and appreciate something in her life every time she noticed she was putting herself down.

The woman sincerely practiced for two days. During that time, she felt her heart open and could sense happiness again. As she continued to practice, her perceptions began to change and her mind started to show her new possibilities. It was as if the sun was coming out after a long, dark, cloudy winter. One month later, her therapist confirmed the change was real and she was able to stop taking drugs.*

When the emotions are back in balance, your mind has a chance to achieve clear common sense. Regular practice of FREEZE-FRAME puts unmanaged emotions in check and wakes up your heart so your mind and emotions can enjoy the clarity and fun of life.

Building Good Emotional Habits

When you're first beginning to build up strength and confidence in a new skill, the least line of resistance has a strong tendency to win out. In other words, you may be inclined to revisit old emotional habits.

As you encounter them, you will become more aware of just how ingrained some of the habits seem to be. You could find yourself saying, "I knew it, FREEZE-FRAME doesn't work." But don't despair.

You formed these habits when you were mostly unconscious of them and saw no alternative. Now you are conscious of them and have a powerful new tool to assist you.

*Depression may have a biochemical basis. Individuals should consult their physician regarding feelings of depression or concerning medication.

Once you genuinely build strength by your own practice, it's yours—an acquired skill that can be relied on and developed more and more. It's the power to have *choice* in how you want to mentally and emotionally react to life's situations, which is a gigantic leap forward in dissolving your own stress deficit. As you practice FREEZE-FRAME, you'll build a new habit of increasing the distance between you and your old emotional habits.

The Power of Neutral

Chapter 6

CHAPTER HIGHLIGHTS

- Finding the Neutral Zone
- Getting to Neutral
- A Time Shift

When you are first learning FREEZE-FRAME, or when you are in an emotionally-charged situation, sometimes the best you can do is to get to neutral. Neutral is where you've disengaged from the disturbance but haven't determined a new direction yet. Simply shifting to neutral can save you a lot of energy.

Mental and emotional balance from the heart is the first step to neutral.

As thoughts and feelings play a major role in everything you do, it is through these elements that you experience your happiness and peace of mind—or the worst day you've ever had.

FREEZE-FRAME is not going to change every unpleasant situation you face. Life will still be life. But it can help you find the neutral zone that can save yourself from being drained and depleted time after time.

Neutral is the safe zone, the place where thoughts and concerns come to rest for a moment or two so you can gain that new level of clarity. When you're in neutral, you can adapt more quickly even if outcomes don't match expectations. With your emotions more balanced, you can be more objective in the moment. For example, you'll find you don't waste energy pre-judging a person or situation, because being neutral keeps judgments at bay so you can uncover a deeper comprehension of what's happening.

Neutral is where you'll find that higher ground in a time of confusion or indecision. It's like the balance point on a seesaw, holding steady between up and down. Reaching neutral consistently builds a deep reserve of inner power.

Neutral is a platform for objectivity in the moment. If you're unable to hold that objective position and find yourself right back in the heat of things, don't give up and think there's no hope. Be patient with yourself. Try to FREEZE-FRAME and find that neutral point again. A method to trigger hope is sticking with it and not panicking at the first difficulty. If you were dealing with a couple of wild kids having a temper tantrum, would you just let them have their way because it was too hard to stop the noise? Similarly, if your emotions and racing mind don't just go away on command, try not to be impatient. Have compassion for yourself just as you would with a child. Use understanding to harness that wild, reactive energy. Each time you try, you exercise that muscle a little more. Soon it becomes fun to see your personal stress deficit being reduced daily.

Neutral is not up or down, good or bad, right or wrong. It's more like wait and see. If you've ever heard two people arguing over opposing opinions, I'll bet your instincts said that if they both would pause to take a sincere look, they'd be more likely to untangle the mess they'd created. If you can see that in others, try to be aware of that process in yourself.

As you gain more control and mastery over emotional reactivity, and increase your skill at shifting to neutral, you'll begin to notice more subtle mind patterns to shift. For instance, let's say you're arguing with a coworker. You have your opinion, they have theirs, and there's tension in the air. Your heart intelligence is telling you that the issue isn't worth the ill-will you're about to generate, but you don't quite listen deeply to yourself because you are justifying your stance with the "significance" of the issue. If you could recognize this and return to neutral by taking the significance out—shifting from your "point" to your heart—you might be amazed at the clarity, perspective and insight you gain, and relationships you keep.

Getting to Neutral

The first two steps of FREEZE-FRAME can help you get to neutral. You recognize that you are feeling stress and shift your focus away from the racing mind or disturbed emotions to the area around the heart. It is extremely simple to do, but don't underestimate its power.

Just the simple act of shifting your attention away from the emotional reaction slows or stops the adrenaline surge and begins to increase the coherence of the information being sent from the heart to the brain. Neutral is a very powerful position to be in. It's like defusing a bomb. Completing the FREEZE-FRAME would give you a wider perspective and intelligent alternatives; but by going to neutral, at least the bomb won't explode. You've stopped the negative drain, the vicious cycle of hurt and react, fight or flight, judge or panic, and in doing so, given yourself a window of opportunity.

A Time Shift

Have you ever wished you could go back and change the way you handled or said something? Many people have experienced this numerous times. But no matter how many times you replay the scene in your mind, you can't change it. It's in the past. All you can do is pick up the pieces and move on.

Consider FREEZE-FRAME as a sort of portable time machine, one that can't literally take you back in time but one that helps wake you up in the moment so you can experience more quality time in the future. Think about all the energy you could save at work, with your family or any other aspect of your life, if you had the power to manage yourself more effectively in the moment when dealing with people or issues.

Practicing FREEZE-FRAME allows you to be more conscious of your feelings and perceptions in the moment. By helping you relinquish what you would have done, it lets you shift to a new option that would be best for you and everyone else involved. Impulsive mental reactions and choices often create time-wasting stress. Of course, you can learn lessons from long, drawn-out, stressful situations but it's not the best way to learn. A more beneficial lesson to acknowledge is that you don't have to keep learning that way.

When you make an efficient choice in moments of indecision, you establish more effectiveness within a given time span, saving energy and stress. That's a time shift. Inefficient choices can literally produce years of stress—a time loss.

Making healthier choices is like preventive maintenance. It helps you unite with what your heart really knows rather than just following what your mind wants because you "can't help it," and later paying the dues. It's a common-sense way of reducing stress and saving energy in your psychological system. This is the same type of common sense as using a crow bar to pull out nails rather than using your teeth. One choice is so much better that the other seems foolish.

Managing the Mind

Chapter 7

CHAPTER HIGHLIGHTS

- Leveraged Intelligence
- Balance
- New Clarity
- Increased Creativity

As you learn to FREEZE-FRAME, your mind will be one of the big winners. People's mental perspectives often cloud their reactions, inducing stress and ineffectiveness. What you want is fresh, clearheaded perception in order to make wise decisions, solve problems creatively and function at your highest mental capacity.

Our image of a good judge in a court of law is one who has acquired the self-control to hear with his heart, not just his head.

What this technique really teaches is that you can either bathe your brain in chaos or you can send it coherent, focused information.

Remember, by "heart," I don't mean emotionalism. I mean intuitive intelligence. The ideal judge uses the two working jointly in balance—head and heart—to clearly see all sides, then put together a summary of his findings. Do you think he could do this with his mind "knowing what it knows"? He has earned his position in life by suspending his opinions so he can take in the whole picture. What about your own inner judge? How balanced can your perspectives be when you are under stress?

As we've shown, FREEZE-FRAME helps increase the coherence in the two-way communication system between the heart and brain and balances the nervous system which regulates heart rate, blood pressure and many other glands and organs. The increased coherence in the heart rhythms allows the cortex (perceptual centers in the brain) to process information more efficiently. This combined with a balanced emotional system allows you to have a more intuitive, balanced perspective in any situation. As you FREEZE-FRAME, you have better access to the information you already have stored in the brain and new solutions provided by the heart can reach the conscious mind. This is critical for effective decision-making.

The mind cannot manage itself. Without meaning to, it often limits itself (and *you!*) by thinking it already knows all there is to know.

In the information age, it's important to remain open and flexible. Data is constantly bombarding us, forcing us through fast-paced changes. As your skill with FREEZE-FRAME increases, your intuitive intelligence will become more active and available, offering the mind valuable new insights it can't construct on its own. In this way, your mind can break out of the boxes it has contrived through what I call "hand-me-down" programs.

These are old mind-sets and thought patterns that limit perception and options. It's hard to let go of these thought patterns because they're comfortable and much of your security has been based on them. It's the lack of self-security that keeps people clinging to old "hand-me-down" mind habits that have proven to be inefficient and ineffective. As you activate the intuition more consistently, you find a deeper security than acquired intellectual knowledge alone brings.

Knowledge is always changing; but wisdom, through the heart-activated intuition, is deeper and wider in its scope. Wisdom gives you the power to handle change at high speed without losing your balance or sense of security.

Leveraged Intelligence

If you're mentally on overload and can't shut off your mind, you may feel you have lost control. And you have. You've become a victim of your own mind. To turn mental stress into an asset, FREEZE-FRAME and shift to neutral. Then listen to your heart to achieve power over mind ramblings. As you act from heart intuition, the mind can shift gears and go in a healthier direction. When you shift an attitude, energy starts to follow in that direction.

People often attempt to think positively without first making an attitude shift and then wonder why nothing changes. This is because attitudes contain feelings and it takes more than a few positive thoughts to reroute the feelings contained in an attitude—especially a negatively-slanted attitude (like resentment or poor self-image). On its own, the mind struggles and usually fails in building attitude shifts without the strength and forbearance of the heart's commitment. Approaching attitude changes from the heart-feeling level makes it easier to secure a lasting shift.

People will achieve more of their personal goals in the future as they truly learn to "put heart into what they do." Freeze-Framing is a window of opportunity to engage your heart feelings in your decision-making. It offers you deeper understanding of issues the mind often overlooks. With practice you can shift gears and produce energy-saving attitude adjustments throughout the day. You gain what I call "leveraged intelligence" with practical applications. It's leveraged intelligence that restrains you from inviting and repeating the same stress patterns that drain your system and dilute your peace. Leveraged intelligence emerges when the mind and the heart share the same "think tank" before taking action.

> ☑ People skilled at FREEZE-FRAME can calm their brain waves each time they use it. Immediately, they heighten their intuitive understanding and increase their power to adapt.

Winning With Heart

With cold hands, cold feet and frazzled nerves, Vicky Tomasino was all alone in her Los Angeles hotel room the night before she was to appear as a contestant on America's #1 game show.

"I'd spent four years on the waiting list after passing the auditions back in New York. Four years! I'd given up all hope, thinking they'd never get around to my name. But the big day was TOMORROW! What was I going to do? I'd never be able to think. I'd make a fool of myself on national TV. I could feel all the blood rushing up to my head.

"Pacing around the room I thought of calling someone, anyone, to help me calm down. OK, I thought, I'll call my daughter. She works at the Institute of HeartMath. She'll be able to tell me how to handle this. 'Dana, help! I'm on tomorrow, and I can't even think!'

"'Don't think,' she said. 'Just ask your heart for the answers.' She said it was better not to force myself to think from my head, but rather to feel intuitively for the right things to say. 'Just have fun! Relax, and stay centered in your heart.'

"The next day it was obvious that the other contestants were really nervous. Meanwhile, I just sat quietly and didn't think about winning. 'FREEZE-FRAME,' I told myself. 'Stop the panic, focus on your heart and ask it to guide you.'

"Finally, it was my turn. I got up and went on to become a 3-day champion and possibly the second highest winner ever on that game show. Why? Because when I asked my heart for the answers, everything began to flow. The words just popped into my head without my thinking of them. It all seemed incredibly easy. I felt surrounded by a positive energy that swept me to victory. With the energy from my heart, I won over $132,000!"

Increasing Clarity

When you're trying to store information, your mind can become so overloaded it ceases to function well. If you FREEZE-FRAME periodically, you can recharge mentally, emotionally and physically, while increasing memory retention and comprehension.

A real estate agent was studying for an exam that would allow him to advance his career. He described how Freeze-Framing helped him retain what was critical. As he pored over reams of data, he was able to absorb information quickly with increased clarity instead of cramming till he was beat. While studying, if you practice this one-minute exercise at the start and again at those points where you begin to feel overloaded, you'll build mental assets and leveraged intelligence.

We've heard numerous examples of students using FREEZE-FRAME to improve test taking. A typical one came from a friend's daughter. She is a good student, but tends to be a perfectionist. On a big math test, she had one problem left to solve just as the recess bell was ringing. She clenched. Then remembered to FREEZE-FRAME and the answer "just popped into my head."

Boosting Creativity

FREEZE-FRAME is more than a tool for managing stress. It's especially useful in enhancing creativity and quality. It calms the mind and emotions and allows for access to intuitive insights. This kind of intelligence is often what people need when involved in a creative process. Creativity itself manifests in a lot of different ways. It's not just about writing a book or a song, inventing a new product or painting a picture. Doing business, raising a family, planning a vacation or communicating in a difficult situation—all require creativity.

A Fortune 100 company was about to announce a merger with another giant in the same industry. The head of Occupational Development had to quickly set up a communication network for the entire global company of over 200,000 employees to insure the smooth flow of information around this major corporate initiative. He had been wrestling with the complexities for some time when he came to a HeartMath business program. After learning FREEZE-FRAME, he decided to use this problem as the subject of one of the heart-focusing exercises.

After five minutes locking into his heart intelligence, he "saw" the insights and gained the clarity he needed for setting up the entire plan. He was very surprised that he was able to clearly envision the whole communication strategy in such a short time span, and that it came to him in such a clear, comprehensive manner.

While the mind alone works incrementally or digitally, heart intelligence can bring in blocks of information at a time.

Using FREEZE-FRAME before engaging in any creative activity activates the benefits of aligning the mind and heart. It yields more intuitive perception at any time. You don't have to wait until you're in stress. Leveraged intelligence multiplies as you apply this technology for intuitive access to all aspects of your life.

With less stress, you have more clarity, more creative ideas.

CREATIVITY ✚ **FREEZE FRAME**

INTUITIVE ACCESS

✚

LEVERAGED INTELLIGENCE

Added Enjoyment and Quality of Life

FREEZE-FRAME WORKSHEET

Pick a situation—either personal or professional—that could use a creative boost. Write down the situation and your most recent ideas about it. Take a couple of minutes to do this.

Project/situation needing creativity/quality boost:

_____

_____

_____

_____

_____

_____

_____

- Shift your focus to the area around your heart. Pretend you're breathing through your heart to help focus your energy in this area. Keep your focus there for 10 seconds or more.

- Reexperience a positive feeling. You can use the same feeling you used before or pick another one.

- Now, using your intuition, common sense and sincerity—ask your heart—what are some creative options for this situation?

- Listen to what your heart intuition says in answer to your question. Stay focused in the heart and write your ideas under "Intuitive Perspective."

Intuitive Perspective:

_____

_____

_____

_____

_____

_____

_____

_____

_____

Enhancing Business Effectiveness

Chapter 8

CHAPTER HIGHLIGHTS

- Putting FREEZE-FRAME to work
- Opportunities in Crisis
- Efficiency Boost: Time Savings
- Stress in Business

"The background physiology and the scientific underpinning of this technique are absolutely sound, which is why we went ahead with pilot studies at Shell. I don't think the science is new, but getting it to work with individuals—and particularly technical people—is!" [1]

Graham Bridgewood, M.D., Chief Medical Officer, Shell International

Business needs more heart. I could cite statistic after statistic of how many people in business feel treated like cogs, not people, of how uncared for they feel, and how unmotivated and unproductive they are as a result.

The number of workers feeling highly stressed has doubled since 1985 to 46%. Business is changing rapidly and it's harder and harder to stay competitive. Companies that treat people better and put heart in what they do will have the real competitive advantage in the future.

Business guru, Tom Peters, author of the books *In Search of Excellence* and *Liberation Management,* seems to agree:

"Store shelves groan under the weight of new products, but few have heart. Service offerings are about as lifeless. Most hotels, for example, spent the last decade buffing their customer service. The mechanics are better. Bravo. But the heart is usually absent: the sincere sense of 'Welcome to my home' as opposed to 'I've gotta remember to act like I care.'"[2]

It's the lack of heart that's gotten business where it is today, with more stress and anxiety than ever. People are frying by the truckloads. Every day countless numbers hate to go to work; their hearts are not there. FREEZE-FRAME activates the power of your heart to guide you in directions where business can become more successful and satisfying.

Because business today is so fast-moving, it takes tremendous energy to keep up without getting eaten up. Business involves head thoughts, head decisions, being in your head all day long with many people winding up with a headache.

As you experience for yourself how fast this simple, powerful tool releases stress on the inside, you'll find it a work tool as essential as your computer.

Even at the highest level of global corporations, there is a growing awareness of the need for tools to help individuals unfold their intelligence and fulfillment—and the bottom line business reasons for doing so.*

Increasing the overall awareness, effectiveness and intelligence of the individual leads to measurably healthier organizations.

From Chaos to Coherence, which I just coauthored with HeartMath vice president Bruce Cryer, is a complete discussion of the HeartMath application to business and organizational life.

Business Stress Check

Which of these business-related stresses apply to you?

☐ Overloaded with deadlines

☐ Always rushed

☐ Communication conflicts with coworkers

☐ Need stress or pressure to get the job done

☐ Unappreciated for your efforts

☐ Consumed by work issues after hours

☐ No job security

☐ "Overcaring" —getting close to burnout

Maximizing Business Potential

As increasingly large numbers of businesses have begun to use this technique in the workplace, our understanding of the practical applications of FREEZE-FRAME has grown. Feedback from these professionals indicates that, above and beyond the personal health benefits they receive, their enhanced performance is having a measurable impact on the companies' overall productivity. Companies are saving money. Customer relations have improved. Interoffice conflict has diminished while teamworking is enhanced. And overall stress is idling at a much lower level than ever before.

Putting FREEZE-FRAME to Work

HeartMath corporate clients— such as Motorola, Hewlett-Packard, Royal Dutch Shell, Cathay Pacific Airways, and Boeing—have experienced the value of heart intelligence—the synergy of intellectual, intuitive and emotional intelligence—in increasing individual and organizational performance and health.

A client of ours is one of Canada's largest banks. With a strong commitment to learning, it trained over 1300 employees in FREEZE-FRAME over a one-year period. The bank had 5 internal trainers certified to teach the FREEZE-FRAME technique, who then delivered seminars to employees representing a cross-section of position, age, background and education. A sample of employees was surveyed six to eight months after the FREEZE-FRAME training to determine the extent of their use of FREEZE-FRAME and the self-assessed effects of the technique on behavior, health and overall well-being.

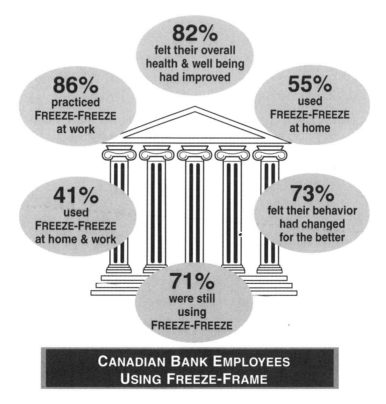

82% felt their overall health & well being had improved

86% practiced FREEZE-FREEZE at work

55% used FREEZE-FREEZE at home

41% used FREEZE-FREEZE at home & work

73% felt their behavior had changed for the better

71% were still using FREEZE-FREEZE

CANADIAN BANK EMPLOYEES USING FREEZE-FRAME

The word has spread, and by early 1998 over 2,500 bank employees have participated in FREEZE-FRAME and IQM (Inner Quality Management) programs.

Escaping from Stress

Increasingly, business is becoming "lean and mean." This translates into more pressure, longer work hours, increased responsibility and the need to adapt quickly to change. For most, the threat of corporate downsizing is present as well. These external pressures, combined with a lack of mental and emotional self-management, can result in the slow burn of accelerating stress. Yet, as the statistics in Chapter 1 show, many people are unaware of the seriousness of their inner stress until they come to the end of their rope—in mental, emotional or physical burnout.

Does this sound familiar? You wait all year for a one or two-week vacation to escape from stress, only to discover that the stress travels with you. Just getting away from the job and the usual routine can be stressful. Then for the first few days of the vacation, it's hard to turn off the mind and unwind. For the next several days you begin to feel like you're on vacation. But as the vacation draws to a close, problems or pressures back at the office or at home start to intrude again in your thoughts. The last few days you're restless with these concerns. When you return to work, you wonder what happened to your vacation.

Freeze-Framing won't extend your vacation or change the demands of your job, but it can release much of the built-up pressure so that you can enjoy your holiday.

Seeing an Opportunity in Crisis

Vivian Wright is an internal consultant and certified FREEZE-FRAME and IQM trainer for one of the world's largest and most successful computer and electronics companies. Recently, at the completion of some intensive travel, Vivian agreed to attend a short planning session for a worldwide organization design conference being held the following week. She was looking forward to the next few days in her office and at home to clear her desk and her head when she heard the news: one of the two conference organizers had to withdraw. This left her colleague, Peter, stranded in a phase of design new to him. Now Vivian's help was needed.

"I wanted to go home and unwind. The last thing I wanted was another week on the road," Vivian admitted, "but what could I do? A worldwide team of 45 people expected a breakthrough. I Freeze-Framed for a minute and shifted gears fast."

Vivian and Peter faced the task of creating a plan for the conference. "I knew I had to make this thing happen," Vivian recalls. "I had expert knowledge, but I was overwhelmed with the details. What would really help the team? Where would the leverage points be? How could I be truly effective and avoid massive stress?"

Peter was also familiar with the FREEZE-FRAME process, and suggested they both apply the technique to get key insights on how to make smart and efficient choices. After doing a FREEZE-FRAME together, they synthesized their ideas and wrote them down. Now their task seemed achievable and simpler. "We spent another thirty minutes outlining our next steps and felt prepared for the meeting."

On Monday, Vivian recalls, "At one point things got a little fuzzy and we suggested a break. Peter and I left the room. We went outside and Freeze-Framed, leaning against the building. We got the same insight and found that it seemed to fit perfectly with what the others had concluded during the break. We were clearer about how to customize the design process. Everything went very well throughout the conference. As a team, Peter and I were in sync. Our plans and insights were right on track. Just before a pivotal design section the second afternoon, I taught everyone how to FREEZE-FRAME. Teams worked through critical areas of design with apparent ease and the background hum of tension disappeared. The high quality of dialogue and work was evident."

Vivian remembers how different the flip charts were after the FREEZE-FRAME, "They weren't as messy and looked more like the diagrams of engineers!"

"The energy was really high at the end of the conference," Vivian recalls. "I went home feeling like a million bucks. Instead of exhaustion, I felt a glow of gratitude. I had helped a friend and colleague, rose to a challenge, and helped create a successful, productive, and healthy two days for 45 people under pressure. We turned stress into success."

Efficiency Boost: Time Savings

Sometimes people say to me, "It sounds like a great idea, but I'm a busy professional. There just aren't enough hours in the day—I don't have time for this!"

The reality is, you save time and energy when you FREEZE-FRAME. When you slow down, step back a moment and put things in perspective, you can then move on with more efficiency. It only takes a moment to adapt and control how you respond. Managing your energy is not a foreign idea or unrealistic possibility. It's accessible.

Let's say you're a busy executive and a single parent. You have the usual pressures at work, compounded by the daily juggling act of your kids' after-school activities, managing the household, errands to run, bills to pay, meals to make, clothes to wash. The list seems endless. One morning you wake up late; finding yourself late would be your first chance to exercise your

FREEZE-FRAME muscle that day. But you say, "Being late for work is a real problem. I *need* to get upset over that. I could lose my job, my kids will starve." It's so tempting to justify allowing the mind and emotions to have control over you.

Then your heart reminds you of the efficiency of taking a moment to FREEZE-FRAME, but your mind interrupts with, "But I ... really ... am ... late! I don't have time to FREEZE-FRAME. I need to go fast and don't have time to stop." So you race around to get ready, your mind churning over all the things that could go wrong if you show up late again.

Here's an opportunity to take a deeper look now—inside yourself. Getting upset, irritated and frustrated over being late will not change the outcome, except perhaps to make it worse. But grabbing a moment to FREEZE-FRAME and realizing that you've got to handle this—one way or another—might provide you with the extra edge to collect yourself and move in a more efficient manner without the stressful repercussions.

So instead, you race out of the house forgetting your files for that important business meeting. Now you're really in trouble because the client will see you as scattered and unprepared. There you are, at your desk, frustrated and judging yourself for being so stupid. If you had stopped for one minute and Freeze-Framed, you would have gained enough inner balance to step back and make sure you had everything you needed before you left the house. You would have arrived a little later, but you would have been prepared—and saved yourself from draining your mental and emotional accumulators.

Creative Resistance vs. Stress

Many people believe that stress is a necessary motivator for business success. If adrenaline isn't constantly pumping through them and everyone else, they think the job won't get done. It's critical to know the difference between what I call *creative resistance*, which recharges your batteries, and the stress that drains and ages you.

As science has shown, stress reactions cause the release of hormones that can be energizing and fun in the moment, but can also deplete and damage the human system in the long run. Stress reactions inhibit cortical function, and therefore clear, productive thinking. Example: You're in the midst of a key strategy session, but a long-standing conflict with a coworker attending the meeting is starting to boil over. At first, the tension feels stimulating, but its biological consequences prevent any creative decisions being reached, so you finally leave the meeting without completing the task. An hour later, once your emotions calm down, the key strategies become clear. FREEZE-FRAME would have allowed you to shift perspective and generate coherent heart rhythms, facilitating cortical function for the clarity your needed (in the moment).

The goal is to maintain balance while you exert yourself—and know when to stop. It's fun stress, like stretching yourself to jog that extra mile without pushing yourself over the edge. Your nervous system remains in balance, releasing regenerative hormones throughout your body and transforming stress into available, productive energy.

To be able to think on your feet with both your heart and your head alleviates considerable stress. Remember, you want to create balance in the two-way communication system between your heart and your brain. This leads to a greater ratio of peace to stress and much more fun. Many in business now understand that giving attention to overcare and stress is at the hub of better business. Coherent attention paid to these areas is the foundation of business effectiveness and will lead to greater harmony between business and people.

In business today you can FREEZE-FRAME frequently to great benefit. You can utilize it at every turn—when you're feeling rushed or overloaded; in the middle of a communication conflict; when you're overcaring about a client or the impending quarterly financial report; when your boss ignores your sincere efforts, *again*; when thoughts about work keep consuming you at home or with your family; and especially if you're feeling burned out.

Many of the external issues in business that cause stress will not change overnight, but each time you shift your perspective you achieve more personal power to adapt and come out ahead. With practice, this new perspective becomes automatic and a way of life. It will help you adapt to what you can't change and help you see solutions for what you can change. It feels good to experience the flex of your own empowerment and keeps your system filled with hope. Heart works.

"I was one of those who thought I didn't have time to take a class in FREEZE-FRAME. But after looking at the project I was about to start and seeing it would take who-knows-how-many hours, I decided to go to the class just to take a break. It turned out to be one of the most useful classes I have ever taken. Using the techniques, I went back and successfully completed a difficult design project in just under an hour!"

Design Engineer, Boeing

Empowering Relationships

- Improved Relationships
- Dealing with Heartbreak
- Balanced Care vs. Overcare
- Managing Family Stress

You can build strong, loving connections to others only when you have a strong, loving connection between your own heart and mind.

Glen and Jenny were at the end of their rope. After 7 years of marriage, they still fought about things they'd disagreed on from the very first day. No matter how much they wanted to save their relationship and honor their commitment to one another, they couldn't seem to shake the resentment that had built up between them. If ever a marriage was on the rocks, it was theirs. As a last ditch effort, they sought out the help of a psychologist.

Rather than asking the couple to face each other, fully armed with years of complaints, and fight it out, she offered them a new approach. In the first session, Glen and Jenny learned the basic steps of FREEZE-FRAME.

Every time the hurt, resentment or blame came up, they practiced the technique. If one of them started to argue, they both took a FREEZE-FRAME time-out to access their heart intuition for direction and listen to it. In those moments, they each became very quiet and introspective. It was as if a veil had lifted, giving them new insights. Glen began to notice that every time he accused Jenny of not understanding him, his strongest feelings were attached to old memories he had carried around since childhood—not to anything Jenny had done. And after a few minutes of FREEZE-FRAME, Jenny could admit that she knew Glen loved her, even though she accused him of not caring. Gradually, their perceptions of each other began to change. They found their heightened intuition offered them surprising new options.

Within the first few days, the bouts of arguing defused. Their relationship began to improve. At the following therapy session, each one admitted they were the one—not their partner—who was perpetuating the war. By seeing how they were each contributing to the problem, they cut out blame and focused on changing their own reactions instead of trying to change one another. After a few weeks, they began reexperiencing moments of the love and appreciation they felt when they first were married.

FREEZE-FRAME helps to access balance and power within you so you can

> ☑ FREEZE-FRAME helps to access balance and power within you so you can approach your relationships more effectively.

approach your relationships more effectively. In the process, you begin to communicate more authentically and sincerely. Instead of draining the love out of your relationship through overcare and expectations, you learn to nurture the true love and care. A harmonious relationship with one you love can enhance your work, health and entire well-being.

But when it's not working, a relationship can be a massive merry-go-round of overcare and stress. Jealousy, envy, fear of rejection, sexual frustration and loneliness can dramatically sap your personal vitality. Many people don't think of these insecure feelings as stress but they can have serious health consequences and take an enormous toll on your well-being.

Whether you are single, married or divorced, relationship issues can become so sticky or problematic, some leveraged intelligence is required. If you're stuck mentally and emotionally in relationship stress, you can begin to feel the whole thing's not worth it—that the conflict and pain you feel when you're in a relationship outweighs the loneliness you felt without one!

When the Other Person's Not Changing

Here's a common objection to watch for in relationships. You are in a tense conversation. You are Freeze-Framing and managing to stay neutral, but the other person keeps right on hammering his point with no regard to how fair you're playing. It would be so easy to lose your cool, to think, *"Well, if he's not going to listen, why should I? I'm not changing until he does!"*

Life is not going to transform around you every time you FREEZE-FRAME. So be prepared. On the other hand, don't ignore how much your balanced attitude can affect the people and situations you face. Appreciate yourself for the efforts you make, regardless of the outcome. If you maintain inner balance in any given situation, whatever others do, you are properly taking care of your own self. That's okay to do, and an intelligent choice.

FREEZE-FRAME helps you keep alive the original care and love in your relationship by not dowsing it with stress. It allows you to step back from anger or insecurity in the moment, find a deeper heart perspective and build an inner net of understanding between you.

Balanced Care vs. Overcare

Overcare is one of the most consequential energy drains in the human system. Instead of enhancing your life and relationships, it actually keeps you from enjoying the people and things you care about.

True care enriches relationships. But if care crosses the line into worry or anxiety, it becomes overcare. Emotions build until you're just as tangled up in them as if you were lost in an argument.

Most people assume that feelings in the heart cause overcare. They don't. The unmanaged mind puts people into overcare. The heart cares, but it's the mind that builds up worry and anxiety. This creates constant, low-grade stress and can eventually lead to burnout of

Relationship Stress

Which of these relationship stresses do you experience?

- ❏ Conflict
- ❏ Disappointment
- ❏ Insecurity
- ❏ Social frustration
- ❏ Jealousy
- ❏ Inability to communicate
- ❏ Loneliness
- ❏ Sexual frustration
- ❏ Loss
- ❏ Discontentment

yourself and your relationship. Even if you don't reach this point, living in overcare can still feel like you're flying on a plane with one engine out.

Balanced care is regenerating. As you've read in Chapter 3, feelings of care induce harmonious, coherent heart rhythms which align the nervous system, enhance the immune response and help mental clarity. Overcare, on the other hand, causes stress-producing heart rhythms, creating out-of-sync signals between the heart and brain, impairing decision-making ability, lowering the immune response and your personal energy level as well.

Dr. Anne Berlin, a San Diego psychologist and certified FREEZE-FRAME trainer, says, "Many of the women I see in my practice are involved in overcare. By the time they get to me, they feel drained. Some are having panic attacks or anxiety, waking up in the middle of the night, overcaring about something that they didn't resolve during the day. These women need help before they break down with anxiety or depression. I've been using FREEZE-FRAME with many of my patients. 40% experience some immediate relief in the first session. If they continue to practice FREEZE-FRAME, another 30% begin experiencing relief within four sessions. They're able to calm themselves down, regulate their heart rhythms, increase their energy, and they love it because they feel more in control."

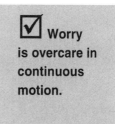

Worry is overcare in continuous motion.

An onslaught of worries about your children, jobs, traffic, sports, pets, relationships, life and everything can occupy a tremendous amount of energy throughout the day. People are especially prone to justify overcaring in relationships and job issues. Yet you can damage yourself far more from overcare than you can by losing a relationship or a job. It's like a social predator that preys on the mental and emotional nature, producing serious energy drains both in individuals and in the collective environment.

The deceptive aspect of overcare is that it can always be justified by the mind. Worry and overcare seem natural, but they're really "hand-me-down" stressor patterns from uneducated social belief systems. A little worry is hard to prevent at times, but with practice you can minimize it and save your health and happiness. Science has already proven that worry takes its toll. Take it out of your diet plan; it's loaded with unhealthy additives. I know from experience.

Overcare in relationships leads to attachments that smother people's spirits and eventually alienate those with whom you are trying to get closer. Care for people, but don't put a noose around them. That just creates emotional luggage which drags them down until, finally, for self-preservation, they free themselves from that luggage and release their spirit to enjoy life again. Simply said, unbalanced care for people prevents them from being themselves. People don't like that. You don't. Freeze-Framing helps you become more conscious of energy drains from overcare.

Overcare occurs when there is mental or emotional over-identity with people, opinions, attitudes, issues, results. People often recognize the energy depletion and strike out in anger at others, or become angry with themselves for being victimized by their own overdoing. Still, due to lack of self-management, they continue the overcare, accumulating further stress while staying trapped in that same feedback loop.

Overcare can be a hard momentum to reverse. Preventive maintenance would be a wise energy investment. How do you know if overcare is sapping your vitality? Look at the people and issues you care about. Is your caring in a given area causing stress? If you find yourself feeling drained because of care, that's an excellent time to FREEZE-FRAME the situation and take a deeper look to see if it's overcare rather than care. While Freeze-Framing, ask yourself, "Is my caring helpful for myself and others? Or is it draining both myself and others?" Remember, balanced care is regenerative; overcare is depleting. If you're honest with yourself, your heart intuition and common sense will broaden the perspective and assist you in attaining balanced care.

It takes a little practice to observe and understand the fine line between care and overcare. If you're in a traffic jam and running late, it's normal to care about it. However, if you don't keep the care in balance, it transforms into anxiety, dilutes your energy reserve and can ruin the rest of your day. Freeze-Framing hands you a chance to put your outgoing energies of overcare in check now, in order to save pain and stress "backwash" later.

> ☑ Remember, balanced care is regenerative; overcare is depleting...It takes a little practice to observe and understand the fine line between care and overcare.

Observe yourself for a week in areas of life that you care about. See if you are manufacturing more stress for yourself or others due to overcare. I think you'll discover this exercise to be fun, interesting and save you time and energy. After you intercept your overcare, then Freeze-Framing will afford you a choice in the moment to prevent an overdraw on your energy account. Peace and quality of life depend on how wisely people spend their energies day-to-day. Why sleep at night to recharge if you're going to squander the energy the next day through mismanagement?

FREEZE-FRAME WORKSHEET

FREEZE-FRAME Practice—Care & Overcare

1. Pick a current issue that you tend to overcare about and write down a brief description below under "Overcare." This could be a personal, relationship, family, work or social issue.

2. Where it says "Head Reaction," write down what you've been experiencing (worry, anxiety, frustration). What have you been going through with this issue?

3. Now, FREEZE-FRAME:

   - **Take a time-out from your overcare issue.**
   - Shift your focus to the area around your heart. Pretend you are breathing through your heart to help focus your energy in this area. Keep your focus there for ten seconds or more.
   - Recall a positive, fun feeling and attempt to reexperience it.
   - Now, using your intuition, common sense and sincerity—ask your heart, what would be a more efficient response to the situation, one that will minimize future stress?
   - Listen to what your heart says in answer to your question.

4. When you are ready, write down your heart's response under "Intuitive Perspective."

Overcare:

_____

_____

_____

Head Reaction (worry, etc.):

_____

_____

_____

Intuitive Perspective:

_____

_____

_____

_____

_____

_____

_____

Losing a Relationship

Relationship loss can be one of the most traumatic human experiences. Some people never recover. According to *The Language of the Heart*, by Dr. James Lynch, "The expression broken heart is not just a poetic image for loneliness and despair but is an overwhelming medical reality."[1]

Lack of human companionship, chronic loneliness, social isolation or the sudden loss of a loved one is one of the leading causes of premature death in America.

Dr. Lynch identified a relationship between loneliness and virtually every major disease, including cancer, pneumonia and mental disease. Appropriately enough, the connection was particularly clear in heart disease—although many heart patients were strangely oblivious of a feeling of loneliness. It was as if they had been disconnected from their own emotional pain.

Astounding as it seems, Dr. Lynch could not help but conclude that "evidently millions of people are dying—quite literally—of broken hearts..." But there is hope. Although the physical heart is indeed taxed when your heart has been broken, the road to recovery does not have to be long and arduous.

A broken heart starts with broken mental and emotional attachments and expectations. Feelings of rejection, hurt and disappointment have gotten mixed in with the real love you felt. The mind replays the hurt over and over, magnifying the pain so it feels like your heart is broken and all love is lost. FREEZE-FRAME can help you extract the real love from the hurt and pain and reopen your heart. With use you can reclaim your own power and gain new hope for the future.

One of the biggest challenges in a relationship occurs when one person wants to move on and the other clings to the relationship. If you're the one clinging, it can feel like the world is caving in and all hope for fulfillment is lost. Your entire self feels like life has turned against you; there is an empty place inside that no one can fill except the one who doesn't seem to care anymore. You've become a victim of your own dependence on another person's "batteries." How could something as simple as FREEZE-FRAME help?

If there were ever a time to turn to your heart power for help, it's now. The paradox is that it seems like your heart is broken, so how could it mend itself? And at those times, if you attempt to go to your heart, you just feel pain. What do you do?

Many people retreat into loneliness after a relationship loss closes their heart. Reopening the heart is essential to the recovery process. Freeze-Framing can speed up that recovery time and help open the next chapter of your life. When people drift away from each other in a relationship, it's hard to re-bridge the gap without first bridging the gap between one's own heart and mind. By attempting that, new hope is often born.

In today's lifestyle, people don't have time for long drawn-out therapy. Things are moving too fast and most can't afford it anyhow. Many relationship breakups could be spared if people deepened the connection between their own hearts and minds. Freeze-Framing helps each partner make that inner connection within themselves first, then with each other. Shallow, veneer communication creates most of the stress deficit in individuals, relationships, businesses, communities and society. People have to earn their way out. Learning to manage the mind and emotions is a profitable place to start. Using FREEZE-FRAME hands you a convenient mirror for self-review.

While loneliness puts your heart at risk, we now know, and have shown in the lab, that feelings of love and care can be self-generated, making you less vulnerable to the health risks associated with loneliness. The more consistently you remember to shift to the heart for comfort and care, the quicker feelings of loneliness can fade, and you can build the inner-magnetics that attract new relationships into your life.

Family Relationships

FREEZE-FRAME is also a great tool for enriching family life. Its simplicity lends itself to all ages and a variety of family scenarios. It can provide a moment of peace to insure smooth transitions: from one activity to the other, work or school to home, at bedtime. It helps parents and children to discriminate intelligent choices from emotional impulses, to resolve conflicts and maintain healthy discipline boundaries.

David and Jenny Pendleton, HeartMath trainers from Great Britain brought their two daughters with them to HeartMath during their certification. While David and Jenny attended the seminar, Emily (12) and Katy (10) learned how to FREEZE-FRAME from the HeartMath child care counselor.

Emily and her family continue to practice and function as a support team for each other, reminding each other—and themselves— to use the tool to get back to normal when things get a bit out-of-kilter. Her younger sister recently called from an overnight at a friend's, feeling a bit homesick. Her mom suggested she FREEZE-FRAME, allowing Katy to comfort herself and let go of her sad feelings.

When Emily has an argument with a friend from school and can't stop thinking about it, she uses FREEZE-FRAME to take her mind off it. She also uses it when worried or anxious. For instance, while in the waiting room for an acting exam, she was feeling very anxious, so she Freeze-Framed and "wasn't at all nervous and did really well."

Emily attends a girl's boarding school near her home and tells this story: "I was in the dorm and my friend was going through a bit of trouble. She's a boarder (Emily's a day student), and was not happy. She doesn't have many friends and misses her parents. So I said, 'Try this, it's what I do to not be agitated.' As I was going through the steps, and she was beginning to feel better, it got really quiet in the room—all the other girls were listening. One of them had been trying to get to sleep. She was listening to me and thought she'd give it a go. All of a sudden this big smile came across her face and she said, 'Wow, it really works.' She had pictured herself doing a really good part in hockey, and that means a lot to her. The next day everyone was coming up to me and asking, 'can you make me happy?'"

The "Know What You Know" Standoff

A typical conflict that happens frequently between parents and teens is when parents believe they know best and teens believe they know best.

Each "knows what they know" and won't even talk to one another. It's an obvious and all-too-common problem. The consequences of "knowing what you know" and not being open to new perceptions can be seen in the increasing numbers of high school dropouts, runaways and youthful offenders. These problems are evidence of a huge gap between parents, teens and our educational system.

The largest problem, according to teenagers, is that parents (and adults in general) don't listen. At the same time, many parents feel teens don't listen. Using techniques like FREEZE-FRAME, HeartMath facilitates workshops between adults and teens to help improve communication.

In Phoenix, we had an eighth-grade gang member who participated in a FREEZE-FRAME listening exercise with a woman who worked for the school district. It was a pretty surprising interaction. The woman from the school district had grown accustomed to the idea that gangs were "the enemy." She had started to take for granted the lack of communication between gangs and school officials. But when she really turned her attention to the exercise, she was amazed at the sensitivity of this "known troublemaker" and felt tremendous compassion for him. And the boy himself was deeply moved. After the program he went to the vice principal and, with tears in his eyes, told him that this was the first time an adult had ever listened to him. As a result, he found the courage to leave the gang.

Support Systems

Using FREEZE-FRAME in a family, school or work environment is particularly effective when several people are practicing it. This has been most evident in the numerous companies, organizations and schools who have trained an entire staff, department or team in FREEZE-FRAME. We've also seen this in families using the tool and in the many HeartMath "Hubs" (organized study groups) around the country.

When a group of people practice FREEZE-FRAME together, it creates a positive climate of coherent communication, care and support that accelerates the progress of the individuals and empowers the team beyond the sum of the individuals. It helps each person see what would be impulsive reactions and judgments, then presents them with a chance to take more responsible action. The result is individuals learning to be responsible for their own energies and decisions—people who clean up their mental messes before they even make them.

As people utilize this tool together in business, school or family situations, it helps clean up the psychological murk of any relationship environment. Social support has been proven to have beneficial health effects. A study on the effects of love on health published in the scientific journal, *The Annals of Internal Medicine*, found that emotional support dramatically improved survival after a heart attack. Patients who lacked love and care were more likely to die within six months than patients who experienced love and care in their lives. According to the study's author, Lisa F. Berkman, an epidemiologist at Yale University School of Medicine, "There's enough evidence now to say that lack of social support is a risk factor to the heart, similar to high blood pressure, high cholesterol and lack of exercise."[2]

Freeze-Framing promotes maturity through managing mental and emotional energy expenditures in day-to-day relationships and family interactions. Your capacity to do this increases as you sincerely remember to apply the technique.

Sincerity is the amount of heart you focus into a mind intention. For example, a person's intention might be to completely forgive someone and release all the old baggage and resentments. Then, a few days later the same, old, tired judgments and negative feelings pop up again.

What is required for effective change is continuity of sincere effort to release and let go of inefficient thought patterns from the past. Freeze-Framing helps you remember to be sincere in your approach to anything—people, places or issues. Sincerity means a deeper heart commitment to the task.

As I said earlier, heart commitment provides more sustaining power to complete your intention. It assists cleaning out old mental and emotional debris, rewarding you with self-security and esteem. The result is: You feel much better and people around you sense that! As your inner quality improves, the quality of your environment improves. Cleaning up your inner environment is the most supportive gift people can offer to the outer environment.

Our current scientific research is addressing the possibility that living in the aftereffect of stale thoughts and emotions may be far more damaging to people's health than secondhand smoke, hair spray or food additives. You can clean up the air, save the trees and read every dietary label, but until inner mental and emotional rubbish is recycled, there won't be the hope and coherent power necessary to solve the major problems in social consciousness or achieve "wholeness" health. As you learn to manage your inner ecology, you create a new hormonal balance that generates better health and especially inner peace. That's a direct approach to balancing relationships.

Social
Impact

The implications of applying heart intelligence to society's problems are huge. There are solutions, but we can't see them using the same modalities or processes that caused the problems. With both heart and mind, we can build caring communities, design schools that develop children's wisdom and emotional strength along with their intellect and physical strength, and operate institutions with balance, intelligence and appreciation for people and the environment.

The most acute social priority is for individuals to clean up their own mental and emotional messes.

111

Mending Social Stress

Which of these social issues cause you stress?

❑ Financial pressures and uncertainty

❑ Declining social values, in the schools, in the culture

❑ Violence on TV and movies

❑ Pollution, ecological imbalances

❑ Media focus on frightening, negative news

❑ Concerns about child-rearing and family values

❑ Fear of crime, violence or disasters

Inner & Outer Violence

Domestic and social violence usually starts off with a few angry words and a few hurt feelings that don't get resolved, then escalates into feelings of betrayal, rage and revenge. Inner feelings of rage soon spill over into all aspects of society. Social stress multiplies daily with every new report of political upheaval, child abuse, drug abuse, workplace violence, children bringing guns to school, homelessness, ethnic wars or some other crisis.

The root cause of a lot of these social stresses is the inner violence created by dysfunctional communication between the heart and the mind. As social stress increases, we're faced with a choice: Retreat into fear and isolation, become angry and bitter, try to ignore it all, or take responsibility for our own stress reactions. It's how we as individuals handle our seemingly innocent daily stresses that determines our ability to weather the bigger storms.

The most acute social priority is for individuals to clean up their own mental and emotional messes. As people learn how to be responsible for their mental and emotional disarray, new, creative solutions can emerge which will help clean up the social chaos. This can create a foundation for sustaining social change. Whatever most of us have learned about mental and emotional balance, we probably did not learn in school. Rarely does our educational system address the critical issue of mental and emotional self-management. Yet it's a missing link to individual and social peace.

Social Health in Schools

Stress is not restricted to adults. According to the U.S. Social Health Index, conducted by Innovation in Social Policy/Fordham University, America's social health is at its lowest point in 25 years, with young people suffering the most. The index showed kids are more isolated, more pessimistic and have less sense of community. The Children's Defense Fund reveals that over 80% of teens are worried about violence, drinking, guns, sex, drugs and getting a job.

In schools around the country, administrators are beginning to bring FREEZE-FRAME techniques to the classroom to help kids—and the adults who interact with them—find new, healthier ways to communicate and grow.

Kids & Stress

■ In 1940, the top problems in American public schools, according to teachers, were: talking out of turn, chewing gum, making noise and running in the halls. In 1990, teachers identified the top problems as drug abuse, alcohol abuse, pregnancy, suicide and robbery.[1]

■ 20% of the U.S. children haven't had even a ten-minute conversation with a parent in a month.[2]

■ U.S. teen pregnancy rates continue to be among the highest of developed nations; about 1.1 million girls ages 15 to 19 became pregnant in 1991.[3]

113

One of our educational projects involves students at a Florida middle school. The school's counselors noticed that many students were distracted at school by social pressures, anxiety and depression which diverted their attention from focused academic learning, even among students with high ability. So our Education Division was asked to design a course for them that would use FREEZE-FRAME as the foundational tool to help students reduce their stress, keep up their academic focus, improve communication skills and relationships with peers, teachers and family.

This was just what the kids needed. Dramatic gains were measured in areas like anger management, peer empathy, work motivation, parent compliance, leadership skills, locus of control, school attitude and a decrease in the influence of at-risk behaviors. Under the guidance of school counselor Lorie Russell—the project's director—the middle school students are now mentoring 150 first through fifth graders from nearby feeder schools. The program has received a series of state and federal grants, and the school now offers two full-year elective courses, called "Heart Smarts®" and is expanding the program to nearby schools.

Middle School Heart Smarts Student...

"Today in this seminar I really liked the idea of FREEZE-FRAME. I tried it during my history class when this boy was acting really dumb. I felt like hitting him, and then I remembered, and I paused every thought I had and started thinking only about my family and how I loved them and they loved me. I calmed down and smiled. Hitting him just wasn't important. I'm sure this Institute helped the teachers today and will help many more people during the next seminars."

Tony, 13

Middle School Heart Smarts Students:

Thank you for making the program Heart Smarts. It really has helped me a lot, because before I was in a fight with one of my friends, but then I Freeze-Framed. I found out what the problem was and my friend and I both attacked the problem, and now we're best of friends!
— *Jason*

FREEZE-FRAME has really helped me in life. When I get stressed out, I FREEZE-FRAME so I won't do something I'm going to regret. It has helped me prevent situations like an argument with my Mom and a fight with a friend. This is really helpful in life. To tell you the truth, at first, I really didn't believe it worked, yet I proved myself wrong. It does work! Thanks.   — *Terry*

Thank you for your wonderful teachings of Heart Intelligence. It's really helped me with my stress. I appreciate you for caring and knowing that teens get stressed out too. Most people are ignorant to the fact that teens have problems to worry about just like adults. FREEZE-FRAME should be taught to more schools, and maybe the USA won't be so uptight.
— *Mary Beth*

Kids in Treatment

Phyllis Gagnier, HeartMath Independent Certified Trainer and consultant to school districts, tribal communities and private and public organizations shares this story, "I work as a trainer with teachers, parents and children who are highly at-risk. These are kids under court order or having severe problems at home.

"Recently, I met with group of kids and drew a big heart on the board. I said, 'Let's find out what's in our hearts!' One of the boys said there wasn't anything in his heart. So I said, 'Let's just go in there and listen to find out what's there.' To my surprise, he drew a most exquisite flute man and a beautiful flower. It was just gorgeous. Another little girl had drawn beautiful things but then she crossed them out with an X and said there wasn't anything in there.

"The next day I asked, 'What gets in the way of being in your heart?' A boy who had been suicidal started throwing torn up paper in the air. It reminded me of snowflakes surrounding him; it was so beautiful. All of a sudden they were all doing it! There was a free-for-all in the room. Everyone was throwing up paper. It was like a dance. They had never done this before. I felt they had a moment they'd never had before, that they'd felt something spontaneous and rich and very, very beautiful.

"I stayed that evening and watched as they played volleyball. They were getting on each other. I was sitting on the sidelines. There was a certain amount of scuffling and fighting going go. So I called out, 'Is that from your heart? Try that from your heart!'

"One of the kids stopped to reflect for a moment, and then said, 'I'm sorry, that wasn't from my heart.' Then they started monitoring each other and a couple of staff picked up on it. 'Hey! From the heart! Just chill out from the heart.'

"Soon they were playing more like a cohesive team. It was incredible. One of the staff turned to me and said, 'This is the first time they've ever played together like that.' It makes sense, doesn't it? When the kids are in touch with their hearts, they feel good and for a moment, they can let go of feeling bad."

> When the kids are in touch with their hearts, they feel good...

The Information Superhighway

One of the most significant changes in business, government and society today is the growth of the information superhighway. Billions are now being spent on its design and implementation. Industry experts casually envision every home, business, government and institution linked via a vast global information network hooked into everyone's TV or computer. (As of 1998, 100 million people already are linked in such a network.)

Deep concerns have also been raised. What kinds of mischief will computer hackers create? Will there be the equivalent of car jackings on this highway? What about misinformation? Brainwashing? Invasion of privacy? From my point of view, there are two kinds of information highways to be built. One is in "the sky"—high-speed digital networks and satellite uplinks. The other and more important one is in "the street"—in the hearts of people. The latter has to do with the quality of information exchanged between people.

Technology obviously creates many conveniences, but it can also create more complications and complexities for people to keep up with and understand. Stress can be a big problem on the information superhighway—the stress of confused communication, questionable regulation and possibly new forms of technological violence. FREEZE-FRAME is a technology for people to become inner information highway engineers first—the one between an individual's own heart and mind. This highway is a two-way communication system between the heart and the higher perceptual centers of the brain. It is the primary information highway that hasn't been built yet. The global stress deficit is both the evidence and the consequence of that.

Many people today are excited about building networks, but wish they had extra "beef" (more live information that could really help people) to distribute through a network. Building the inner network first will lead to genuine communication between people. This is what can create more coherent, quality communication between businesses, governments and institutions. The completed individual highway will help restore basic peace. Then what goes across the new superhighway can be living information, allowing humanity to realize the full potential of technology.

Money Issues

Financial pressures can create constant anxiety affecting all aspects of life—regardless of your income level. Whether you're barely making your house payments, lost thousands when the oil price dropped, or worry about just feeding your family, anxiety makes it difficult to perceive creative solutions. Anxiety can warp your perspective so you get locked in the mind-set that you will only be happy and secure if you have more money, more gadgets or the latest computer upgrade, a better house, car or job. Even if you have all those things, you can worry about losing them or that your children won't be able to afford to keep them.

Financial pressures can be quite real when bills are due or at tax time, especially if one member of the household has lost a job or you're trying to put your kids through college. These money pressures affect so many diverse things—the time you have for family and friends and the attitudes you hold in raising your children, among others. The Freeze-Framing technique assists your heart in understanding what your core values really are—what you and your family really require for balance and fulfillment—and managing your emotions in the now.

FREEZE-FRAME is not a magic wand that will pay your bills,

provide two months' vacation every year or send your favorite stocks soaring. But it can help you become mentally and emotionally managed while dealing with your current challenges so that you make more intelligent, intuitive decisions—and remember to do what you may already know deep inside.

Dealing with the Unexpected

> ☑ **Here's the social reality today: No matter how hard we try to prevent it, life will still throw us curve balls just when we are not prepared.**

Major changes can happen so fast. One minute you're fine and the next can be a mess. One minute your job is secure, the next minute the company is laying off 15%. One moment you're asleep, the next moment you're picking through the rubble from the earthquake, tornado, flood, fire or hurricane that just rolled through town.

Life is going to be life—meaning, it acts independent of your wishes and preferences. The more you use your heart for security during change, the easier you can approach change as a challenge you can deal with in a healthy way. That's why it's important to establish your values and priorities now. The FREEZE-FRAME technology is designed to assist you in discovering what your values really are and help you remember to live them when the pressure starts to throw you off-kilter. Practicing builds your muscle to release pressure before it accumulates.

How about a backyard story of how even simple social interactions can start out fun, then quickly turn into a mess to clean up later? You're at your next door neighbor Sam's house for a Friday night summer barbecue. It's been a rough week and you're counting on having some fun. You arrive, still a little wound up from work, and before you know it, you make a joke about how long it's been since he mowed his grass, "Why don't you invite some cows over next time, they'd love your lawn!" Sam's offended and tension increases. You think Sam's going a little overboard with his reaction. After all, it was just a joke. You thought you were being funny but nobody laughed.

Well, here is a perfect place to grab FREEZE-FRAME. If you acknowledge what could happen next and step back quickly, you might be able to prevent a mess caused by your faux pas. If not, once he lashes out about how your old car gives a cheap look to the other driveways in the neighborhood and you respond with anger—well, there goes the party. Not only have you messed up a fun time for yourself but you've probably dumped a very wet blanket on everyone else, too.

Through remembering the technique, you can frame that split second bailout, letting your heart intuition direct the next move that takes care of Sam and warms up the party again, preventing much conflict and stress. By chilling out, you can work it out and often avoid the worst case scenarios. Managed reactions save days of energy. This same basic dynamic can happen at a business meeting, a school ground or a political summit conference.

Through the heart you access more of your real spirit and learn to become who you really are. To stay more connected with your heart's intuition would be like a dream come true. Dreams don't have to be pie in the sky. When "sky" comes down to earth and into the street, and as the qualities of spirit are measured

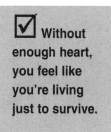

☑ Without enough heart, you feel like you're living just to survive.

in the lab, the solutions to some of our major social stresses may not be so far away. Freeze-Framing aids you in becoming more sensitive to your heart's directive—the power to really change from the inside out.

So take this part to heart, and when you're having one of those talks with yourself, listen deeply to your common-sense thoughts, then act on them and feel the difference. Practice this even a little bit and you'll surprise yourself with what you can accomplish. Whether it's at a party, looking after a friend or a business deal, qualities of love, care, appreciation and especially sensitivity are a breath of fresh air. People are always drawn to anyone with those sincere qualities. They can usually lift the spirits of those around them.

Some are born with a measure of it; some of us need to practice a little more to uncover those qualities. But don't fear; since you have a heart, those qualities are in you. They could just be covered up and need some help getting out. FREEZE-FRAME can, step by step, in any moment in life, help you slow down enough to check in with what your real heart and spirit would do. There is much freedom and stress prevention in learning to be your real self.

The Payoff

The energy you save when you stop and learn to make more effective decisions creates a time shift, whereas an ineffective decision seals you into standard linear time and creates an energy payload deficit of stress and time loss. Freeze-Framing allows you a porthole through which to make an energy-saving time shift.

When dealing with situations, stop and listen more deeply from the heart, then discover how to make attitude adjustments in the moment—meaning *before-the-fact* rather than *after-the-fact.* Attitude adjustments in the moment tame and manage impulsive reactions to people, places and issues.

It's no different than saying to children, "Stop, look and listen before you cross the street." If you really learn to pause, you can weigh out issues consciously rather than reactively. Then, as you tell children, you can look both ways (with head and heart) before moving into an action and its consequences. Sincerity is the key.

> ☑ **Unmanaged reactions to life's situations are a form of sleep-walking.**

Multitudes live for survival and fake their fun. The lack of fun strangles nourishment to your mental, emotional and physical natures. Learning to follow your heart, and balancing the mind's request, replenishes you in a wholeness way, re-activating fun and flexibility, and creating a more active spirit.

The Power of Hope

For millions of people, day-to-day existence feels like an endless treadmill going nowhere fast. For some it's like being lost at sea battling high waves.

Imagine you're adrift in the ocean. You and your partner paddle your life raft for days in search of land. Finally you're both so worn out neither of you can lift the oars anymore. All hope of finding land is lost and you give up. You're lying on the bottom of the boat waiting to die. Then you look up and see a patch of land. Hope! This one drop of hope renews your strength and vitality to vigorously paddle to reach the land, whereas one minute before you were exhausted and dying.

Hopeful thoughts, emotions and attitudes act to refurbish energy levels. Hopeless thoughts and attitudes sap energy and short circuit your capacity to be creative, whether in the workplace or anyplace. People comment, "How can you not have hopeless attitudes if life seems so hopeless?" Many are discovering that following their hearts starts to restore hope in their mental/emotional system. This, in turn, can affect the physical system as a healing tonic and preventive maintenance against many illnesses.

Increasingly, scientific research is confirming the crucial role of positive emotions such as hope in relieving stress and improving health. Yale epidemiologist, Lisa Berkman, Ph.D., also found that positive emotional support alters levels of brain chemicals norepinephrine and cortisol. Although the exact role of those chemicals on the heart is still being investigated, they are believed to affect blood pressure and the heart's response to stress. Leading investigator Jeffrey S. Levin, Ph.D., associate professor of family and community medicine at Eastern Virginia Medical School, compiled over two hundred and fifty published, empirical studies that show statistical relationships between positive attitude, spirituality and various positive health outcomes. According to Levin, while social support is key, a sense of hope and a capacity for forgiveness help people cope more effectively with stress.

Hope for peace and more quality in life is within one's own heart, but without learning to listen to your heart this hope cannot be realized in its completeness. My intention is to provide tools that help people listen to their hearts and actualize hope in practical day-to-day life—in business, social and personal interactions.

Often people's lack of peace and frustration comes from being in their heart consciousness one day, then in their mind consciousness the next day concerning the same issue. Frequently what they think is their mind is their heart and what they think is their heart is their mind. It's hard to know the difference until you stop at each issue to take a deeper look. Freeze-Framing is a simple technology for that in-depth scan, providing a more personal connection with your real feelings rather than your reactive responses.

FREEZE-FRAME is not a magic wand, it's just an opportunity—a chance to listen to your heart in situations. Nevertheless, it's you who has to make the choice to follow your heart. The magic in life comes when you have the power to recognize a heart choice and act on it. As I've said, people suffer from recurring stressor patterns even while their hearts are telling them to make changes. It's the unmanaged mind that represses the heart's promptings, while blaming other people and issues for your continuous misery or lack of peace. As this process continues, it creates hopelessness and despair in different areas of your life.

You can fool others and pretend happiness on the outside, yet on the inside you really know if you feel good and are having a quality life—or not. If you FREEZE-FRAME and listen to your heart more, you change those mind-initiated stressor patterns into self-security and quality within your existing environmental conditions. As you make efforts, yet fall back some, don't beat yourself. Self-beating destroys hope more rapidly than other people can with their comments and attitudes. Self-beating seems justified at the mind level, yet your heart knows that self-judgment only multiplies stress and unhappiness. You can stop that through Freeze-Framing, but don't expect total relief from a single effort.

There is hope to change self-defeating patterns. That hope is within you. As you make attempts toward internal change, you take more of the distortion out of your external relationships. Being true to your heart feelings, you escape much of the stress that comes from the mind running the show. A humor in life is that people fear mind control, yet they're under siege by their own mind's control without the partnership of their heart feelings. It's through heart listening that you learn to become your real self and be free. The heart directs the mind to help create and decorate that achievement.

The new man and woman will be the ones who have learned to follow their hearts and bring their minds into management. As psychology evolves, humanity will realize that real freedom is creating a lasting joint venture and partnership between the heart and the head. Freeze-Framing is a facilitator to help engineer that freedom and create the real paradigm shift—the individual shift—first.

I sincerely hope you have fun and effective results with FREEZE-FRAME. This process is within you by nature. Our system is only a facilitator to help you recall and use the power of your own heart discrimination. The strength and hope you are looking for is also within you; it just needs to be dusted off and oiled on occasion. People get so involved in taking care of the externals in life, they forget to take care of their own mental and emotional self which is where your real peace, quality and fun is registered. So "taking care of self" (inner self) is productive— and it's cost-effective. I can wholeheartedly tell you, "Just practice FREEZE-FRAME and the results will find you."

—The Doc

Endnotes

Introduction

1. Paul J. Rosch, M.D., "Job Stress: America's Leading Adult Health Problem," *USA* magazine, May 1991
2. 1992 United Nations Labor Report cited in Jones and Bartlett, *Stress Management* (Boston, National Safety Council, 1995)
3. Global Burden of Disease and Injury, Harvard School of Public Health, 1996
4. Northwestern National Life - survey.
5. Reuters study
6. *Time* magazine
7. Dr. Bruce McEwen, Rockefeller University, NYC
8. Center for Corporate Health, Beth Israel Deaconness Medical Center, Harvard University.

Chapter 1

1. Some of the physiological information in this chapter is based on the work of Dr. Redford Williams, chairman of the Dept. of Behavioral Science at Duke University. His book, *Anger Kills* (Times Books) explains the stress response in detail.
2. T. Allison et al. Mayo Clinic Proc. 1995; 70(8)
3. New England Journal of Medicine (1998; 338: 171-178)
4. M. Mittleman et al. Circulation. 1995; 92(7)
5. L. Kubzansky et al. Circulation. 1997; 95(4)
6. R. Rosenman. Integr Physiol Behav Sci. 1993; 28(1)
7. World Health Report, 1997
8. American Heart Association: 1998 Heart and Stroke Statistical Update.
9. World Health Report, 1997
10. Archives of Family Medicine (1997; 6:43-49), Dr. Bruce Jonas et al
11. Eysenck HJ. Personality, stress and cancer: prediction and prophylaxis. *Br J Med Psychol.* 1988;61(Pt 1)):57-75.
12. I. Kawachi et al. Circulation. 1994; 89(5).

Chapter 3

1. *American Druggist.* 1994 February issue.
2. Armour J and Ardell J. eds. *Neurocardiology.* 1994, Oxford University Press: New York, NY.

3. Tiller W, McCraty R, and Atkinson M. Cardiac coherence; A new non-invasive measure of autonomic system order. *Alternative Therapies.* 1996;2(1):52-65.

4. American Heart Association: 1998 Heart and Stroke Statistical Update.

5. Armour J. Anatomy and function of the intrathoracic neurons regulating the mammalian heart. In: Zucker I and Gilmore J, *Reflex Control of the Circulation.* Boca Raton: CRC Press, 1991: 1-37.

6. Barrios-Choplin B, McCraty R, and Cryer B. A new approach to reducing stress and improving physical and emotional well being at work. *Stress Medicine.* 1997;13:193-201.

7. McCraty R, Atkinson M, Tiller WA, *et al.* The effects of emotions on short term heart rate variability using power spectrum analysis. *American Journal of Cardiology.* 1995;76:1089-1093.

8. Williams R. *Anger Kills.* New York: Times Books, 1993.

9. Yeragani VK, Pohl R, Balon R, *et al.* Heart rate variability in patients with major depression. *Psychiatry Research.* 1991;37:35-46.

10. McCraty R, Atkinson M, Tomasino D, *et al. The Electricity of Touch: Detection and measurement of cardiac energy exchange between people.* in *The Fifth Appalachian Conference on Neurobehavioral Dynamics: Brain and Values.* 1996. Radford VA: Lawrence Erlbaum Associates, Inc. Mahwah, NJ.

11. Kerr DS, Campbell LW, Applegate MD, *et al.* Chronic stress-induced acceleration of electrophysiologic and morphometric biomarkers of hippocampal aging. *Society of Neuroscience.* 1991;11(5):1316-1317.

12. McCraty R, Barrios-Choplin B, Rozman D, *et al.* New stress management program increases DHEA and reduces cortisol levels. *Integrative Physiological and Behavioral Science.* 1998.

13. Childre, D., *Cut-Thru: How to Care without Becoming a Victim,* 1996, Planetary Publications, Boulder Creek, CA

14. McCraty R, Atkinson M, Rein G, et al. Music enhances the effect of positive emotional states on salivary IgA. *Stress Medicine.* 1996;12:167-175.

15. McCraty R, Barrios-Choplin B, Atkinson M, *et al.* The effects of different types of music on mood, tension and mental clarity. *Alternative Therapies in Health and Medicine.* 1998;4(1):75-84.

16. Rein G, McCraty RM, and Atkinson M. Effects of positive and negative emotions on salivary IgA. *Journal of Advancement in Medicine.* 1995;8(2):87-105.

17. Jandorf L, Deblinger E, Neale J, *et al.* Daily vs. major life events as predictors of symptom frequency: a replication study. *J General Psychol.* 1986;113:205-218.

18. Zachariae R, Bjerring P, and Zachariae C. Monocyte chemotactic activity in sera after hypnotically induced emotional states. *Scandinavian Journal of Immunology*. 1991;34(7):1-9.
19. Rozman D, Whitaker R, Beckman T, *et al*. A pilot intervention program which reduces psychological symptomatology in individuals with human immunodeficiency virus. *Complementary Therapies in Medicine*. 1996;4:226-232.
20. McClelland DC, Ross G, and Patel V. The effect of an academic examination on salivary norepinephrine and immunoglobulin levels. *Journal of Human Stress*. 1985;11:52-59.
21. McClelland D and Jemmott J. Power motivation, stress and physical illness. *Journal of Human Stress*. 1980;6:6-15.
22. Jemmott J, Borysenko Z, Borysenko M, *et al*. Academic stress, power motivation and decrease in secretion rate of salivary secretory immunoglobulin A. *Lancet*. 1983;I:1400-1402.
23. McClelland DC and Kirshnit C. The effects of motivational arousal through films on salivary immunoglobulin A. *Psychological Health*. 1988;2:31-52.

Chapter 4

1. Mortimer quoted in: Howe, S. Change of Heart. *The Sunday Times of London*, November 17, 1997.

Chapter 8

1. Bridgewood quoted in: Howe, S. Change of Heart. *The Sunday Times of London*, November 17, 1997.
2. Peters, T. *In Search of Exellence*. Warner Books, 1988.

Chapter 9

1. Lynch, J. *The Language of the Heart: The Body's Response to Human Dialogue*. New York: Basic Books, Inc., 1985
2. Berkman LF, Leo-Summers L, and Horwitz RI. Emotional support and survival after myocardial infarction: a prospective, population-based study of the elderly. *Annals of Internal Medicine*, 1992, 117(12):1003-1009.

Chapter 10

1. U.S. Department of Commerce Bureau of the Census, "Pace Of Change."
2. Children's Defense Fund, 1994
3. Journal of American Medical Association.

Glossary

Appreciation. An active emotional state in which one has clear perception or recognition of the quality or magnitude of that to be thankful for. Appreciation also leads to improved physiological balance, as measured in cardiovascular and immune system function.

Autonomic nervous system. The portion of the nervous system that regulates most of the body's involuntary functions, including mean heart rate, the movements of the gastrointestinal tract and the secretions of many glands. Consisting of two branches (the sympathetic and parasympathetic), the autonomic nervous system regulates over 90% of the body's functions. The heart, brain, immune, hormonal, respiratory and digestive systems are all connected by this network of nerves.

Balance. Stability, equilibrium or the even distribution of weight on each side of a vertical axis. Is also used to denote mental or emotional stability.

Cardiac coherence. A mode of cardiac function in which the heart's rhythmic and electrical output is highly ordered. HeartMath research has shown that positive emotions such as love, care and appreciation increase the coherence in the heart's rhythmic beating patterns. During states of cardiac coherence, brain wave patterns have been shown to entrain with heart rate variability patterns; nervous system balance and immune function are enhanced, and the body functions with increased harmony and efficiency.

Care. An inner attitude or feeling of true service, without agendas or attachments to the outcome. Sincere care is rejuvenating for both the giver and receiver.

Cardiovascular system. The system in the human body comprised of the heart and the blood vessels.

Cell. The smallest structural unit of an organism that is capable of independent functioning. A complex unit of protoplasm usually with a nucleus, cytoplasm and an enclosing membrane.

Coherence. Logical connectedness, internal order or harmony among the components of a system. Can also refer to the tendency toward increased order in the informational content of a system or in the information flow between systems. In physics, two or more wave forms that are phase-locked together so that their energy is constructive are described as coherent. Coherence can also be attributed to a single wave form, in which case it denotes an ordered or constructive distribution of power content. Recently there has been a growing scientific interest in coherence in living systems. When a system is coherent, virtually no energy is wasted because of the internal synchronization among the parts. In organizations, increased coherence enables the emergence of new levels of creativity, cooperation, productivity and quality on all levels.

Cerebral cortex. The most highly developed area of the brain which governs all higher-order human capabilities such as language, creativity and problem-solving. The cortex, like other brain centers, continues to develop new neural circuits or networks throughout life.

Cortical inhibition. A de-synchronization or reduction of cortical activity, believed to result from the erratic heart rhythms and resulting neural signals transmitted from the heart to the brain during stress and negative emotional states. This condition can manifest in less efficient decision-making capabilities, leading to poor or shortsighted decisions, ineffective or impulsive communication and reduced physical coordination.

Cortisol. A hormone produced by the adrenal glands during stressful situations, commonly known as "the stress hormone." Excessive cortisol has many harmful effects on the body and can destroy brain cells in the hippocampus, a region of the brain associated with learning and memory.

Emotion. A strong feeling. Any of various complex reactions with both mental and physical manifestations, as love, joy, sorrow or anger. Emotional energy is neutral, attaching itself to positive or negative thoughts to create *emotions.*

Entrainment. A phenomenon seen throughout nature, whereby systems or organisms exhibiting periodic behavior will sync up and oscillate at the same frequency and phase. A common example of this phenomenon is the synchronization of two or more pendulum clocks placed near each other. In human beings, the entrainment of different oscillating biological systems to the primary frequency of the heart rhythms is often observed during positive emotional states. This state represents a highly efficient mode of bodily function and is associated with heightened clarity, buoyancy and inner peace. Entrained teams are those which operate with a higher degree of synchronization, efficiency and coherent communication.

Frequency. The number of times any action, occurrence or event is repeated in a given period. In physics, the number of periodic oscillations, vibrations or waves per unit of time; usually expressed in cycles per second. Human intelligence operates within a large bandwidth of frequencies.

Heart. A hollow, muscular organ in vertebrates that keeps the blood in circulation throughout the body by means of its rhythmic contractions and relaxations. The body's central and most powerful energy generator and rhythmic oscillator. A complex, self-organized, information-processing system with its own functional "little brain" that continually transmits neural, hormonal, rhythmic and pressure messages to the brain.

Heart/brain entrainment. A state in which very low frequency brain waves and heart rhythms are frequency-locked (entrained). This phenomenon has been associated with significant shifts in perception and heightened intuitive awareness.

Heart intelligence. A term coined to express the concept of the heart as an intelligent system with the power to bring both the emotional and mental systems into balance and coherence.

Heart rate variability (HRV). The normally occurring beat-to-beat changes in heart rate. Analysis of HRV is an important tool used to assess the function and balance of the autonomic nervous system. HRV is considered a key indicator of aging, cardiac and overall health.

Hormonal system. A hormone is a substance produced by living cells that circulates in the body fluids and produces a specific effect on the activity of cells remote from its point of origin. The hormonal system is made up of the many hormones that act and interact throughout the body to regulate many metabolic functions, and the cells, organs and tissues that manufacture them.

Immune system. The integrated bodily system of organs, tissues, cells and cell products, such as antibodies, that differentiates "self" from "non-self" within our body and neutralizes potentially pathogenic organisms or substances that cause disease. The organizational "immune system" is built upon the core values known to enhance personal fulfillment and well-being, eliminating the emotional viruses which can permeate and destroy the effectiveness and coherence of the organization.

Inner Quality Management® (IQM). HeartMath's multi-contact, research based program for businesses and organizations. Contains modules on internal self-management, coherent communication, boosting organizational climate and strategic processes and renewal.

Insight. The faculty of seeing into inner character or underlying truth and apprehending the true nature of a thing. A clear understanding or awareness.

Intuition. Intelligence and understanding that bypasses the logical, linear cognitive processes. The faculty of direct knowing as if by instinct, without conscious reasoning. Pure, untaught, inferential knowledge with a keen and quick insight; common sense.

Intuitive intelligence. A type of intelligence distinct from cognitive processes, which derives from the consistent use and application of one's intuition. Research is showing that the human capacity to meet life's challenges with fluidity and grace is not based on knowledge, logic or reason alone, but also includes the ability to make intuitive decisions. HeartMath research suggests that with training and practice, human beings can develop a high level of operational intuitive intelligence.

Nervous system. The system of cells, tissues and organs that coordinates and regulates the body's responses to internal and external stimuli. In vertebrates, the nervous system is made up of the brain and spinal cord, nerves, ganglia and nerve centers in receptor and effector organs.

Neural circuits. Neural pathways consisting of interconnected neurons in the brain and body through which specific information is processed. Research has shown that many of these neural connections develop in early childhood based on our experiences and the type of stimulation we receive. Likewise, even later in life, different neural circuits can either be reinforced or atrophy, depending on how frequently we use them. Specific circuits form and are reinforced through repeated behavior, and in this way both physical and emotional responses can become "hardwired" and automatic in our system.

Neuron. Any of the cells that make up the nervous system, consisting of a nucleated cell body with one or more dendrites and a single axon. Neurons are the fundamental structural and functional unit of nervous tissue.

Neutral. In physics, having a net electric charge of zero. With reference to machinery, a position in which a set of gears is disengaged. In human beings, a state in which we have consciously disengaged from our automatic mental and emotional reactions to a situation or issue in order to gain a wider perspective.

Overcare. The result of care taken to an inefficient extreme and crossing the line into anxiety and worry. Overcare is one of the greatest inhibitors of personal and organizational resilience. It has become so natural that people often don't know they are experiencing it, because it postures itself as care. As individuals learn to identify and plug the leaks in their own personal system caused by overcare, they stop draining energy and effectiveness, personally and organizationally.

Parasympathetic. The branch of the autonomic nervous system that slows or relaxes bodily functions. This part of the nervous system is analogous to the brakes in a car. Many known diseases and disorders are associated with diminished parasympathetic function.

Perception. The act or faculty of apprehending, by means of the senses, the way in which an individual views a situation or event. How we perceive an event or an issue underlies how we think, feel and react to that event or issue. Our level of awareness determines our initial perception of an event, and our ability to extract meaning from the available data. Research is showing that when the mind's logic and intellect are harmoniously integrated with the heart's intuitive intelligence, our perception of situations can often change significantly, offering wider perspectives and new possibilities.

Stress. Pressure, strain or a sense of inner turmoil resulting from our perceptions and reactions to events or conditions. A state of negative emotional arousal, usually associated with feelings of discomfort or anxiety that we attribute to our circumstances or situation.

Sympathetic. The branch of the autonomic nervous system that speeds up the bodily functions, preparing us for mobilization and action. The fight/flight response to stress activates the sympathetic nervous system and causes the contraction of blood vessels, a rise in heart rate and many other bodily responses. This part of the nervous system is analogous to the gas pedal in a car.

Time shift. Used here to describe the time saved when we are able to disengage from an inefficient mental or emotional reaction and make a more efficient choice. Time shifting stops a chain-link reaction of time and energy waste and catapults people into a new domain of time management, where there is greater energy efficiency and fulfillment.

Continue the HeartMath Experience with Books, Tapes and Learning Programs

Now that you've read FREEZE-FRAME...

Here are some "next step" suggestions to help reinforce what you've learned and deepen your experience of heart intelligence.

Freeze-Framer: Emotional Management Enhancer—Interactive software program for individuals, health practitioners and teachers. Watch your heart rhythms improve as you practice FREEZE-FRAME on your PC. Displays your heart rate variability via a fingertip pulse sensor. Contains complete instructions on FREEZE-FRAME and HEART LOCK-IN plus three fun, colorful, heart-driven games. Lose stress as you play.

Heart Zones—Instrumental "designer music" by Doc Childre, composed to facilitate autonomic balance and enhance heart/brain communication. Used in all FREEZE-FRAME trainings. Cassette or CD

The HeartMath Solution—Doc's latest book on unlocking heart intelligence. Teaches HEART LOCK-IN, FREEZE-FRAME and CUT-THRU.

HeartMath Discovery Program—Interactive learning program for individuals and groups. Includes *Heart Zones* CD bound in book. (Official study program for HeartMath Hub Groups—see page 138.) Four audio tapes, 120 lesson guidebook.

To order or request a free catalog of our complete product line
Call 1-800-372-3100
or write to:

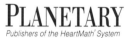

PLANETARY

Publishers of the HeartMath® System

PO Box 66, Boulder Creek, CA 95006
http://www.planetarypub.com

Books by Doc Childre

The HeartMath Solution, coauthored by Howard Martin
CUT-THRU: How to _Care_ Without Becoming a Victim
From Chaos to Coherence, coauthored by Bruce Cryer
Self Empowerment: The Heart Approach to Stress Management
Teaching Children to Love: 80 Games and Fun Activities
A Parenting Manual: Heart Hope for the Family
How to Book of Teen Self Discovery: Helping Teens Find Balance,
    Security and Esteem

Other Books

IHM Research Overview, by Rollin McCraty
Meditating with Children, by Deborah Rozman, PhD
The Hidden Power of the Heart, by Sara Paddison

Books on Tape

The HeartMath Solution Audiobook
FREEZE-FRAME Audiobook
CUT-THRU Audiobook

Scientifically-Designed Music by Doc Childre

Heart Zones: Music Proven to Boost Vitality (Cassette or CD)
Speed of Balance: A Musical Adventure for Emotional & Mental
    Regeneration (Cassette or CD)

Personal Learning Programs

(Includes learning guide with books and/or tapes)
HeartMath Discovery Program
Exploration of the Heart
FREEZE-FRAME Inner Fitness System
FREEZE-FRAME Learning Program w/book or audiobook
CUT-THRU Learning Program w/book or audiobook
Kids' Power Pak
The HeartMath Collection

Activity Tapes for Kids

Buddy Bubbles (Cassette for ages 2-8)
    by Deborah Rozman, Ph.D. and Doc Childre
Heart Signals (Cassette for ages 8-14)
    by Doc Childre and Howard Martin

HEARTMATH®

Retreats and Training Programs

The HeartMath Experience

Individuals from all walks of life interested in personal growth and professional advancement are integrating HeartMath into their lives. These popular training programs are conducted in a variety of social contexts including health care organizations, education, parenting and child development, Fortune 500 companies, personal growth organizations and government agencies.

HeartMath training programs are either held at the IHM training and research facility in Boulder Creek, California or at our customers' sites around the world.

Heart Empowerment

The flagship HeartMath personal development retreat based on *The Hidden Power of the Heart,* by Sara Paddison. Teaches HeartMath tools such as FREEZE-FRAME, Heart Lock-In, Deep Heart Listening, Heart Power Tools to activate higher heart frequencies, Care & Overcare and Heart Mapping®. Overviews of HeartMath's biomedical research, dimensions of intelligence, and blueprints and holograms are presented.

Heart of Wellness

Discover the healing power of the heart. Teaches HeartMath self-management tools, including FREEZE-FRAME, Heart Lock-In, Point Zero, Heart Hologramming and Heart Mapping for healing or health maintenance. Provides a deeper understanding of the heart and its influence on overall health and well-being.

Inner Quality Management

IQM is a three-day, research-based modularized program designed to boost individual and organizational coherence and can be customized to fit an organization's business objectives. Participants learn how to apply HeartMath tools for internal self-management, effective communication, strategic planning, enhancing creativity and decision making.

For more information on trainings and seminars

call 1-800-450-9111

or write to:

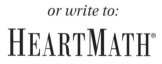

14700 West Park Avenue
Boulder Creek, CA 95006
Visit our web site: http://www.heartmath.com

The Institute of HeartMath

You can contact the Institute of HeartMath (IHM) to start or participate in small study groups (Hub groups) in your area. IHM is a nonprofit organization which conducts scientific research, capital campaigns and the administration of HeartMath Hub programs.

IHM, founded in 1991, specializes in leading-edge research showing the relationship between the heart, mental/emotional balance, cardiovascular function, and hormonal and immune system health. IHM's research has been published in many scientific journals, including *The American Journal of Cardiology* and the *Journal of Stress Medicine*.

For more information
on our research, case studies, Hub groups,
donations or volunteer programs:

Call 831-338-8500

or write to:

INSTITUTE OF HEARTMATH®
A N O N P R O F I T C O R P O R A T I O N

PO Box 1463
Boulder Creek, CA 95006
Visit our web site: http://www.heartmath.org